Medical Library

Queen's University Belfast
Tel: 028 9063 2500
E-mail: med.issue@qub.ac.uk

For due dates and renewals:

QUB borrowers see 'MY ACCOUNT' at
http://library.qub.ac.uk/qcat
or go to the Library Home Page

HPSS borrowers see 'MY ACCOUNT' at
www.honni.qub.ac.uk/qcat

This book must be returned not later
than its due date but may be recalled
earlier if in demand

Fines are imposed on overdue books

Color Atlas of

ORAL MEDICINE

Second Edition

William R Tyldesley

M Mosby-Wolfe

Copyright © 1994 Times Mirror International Publishers Limited
Published in 1994 by Mosby–Wolfe Publishing, an imprint of Times Mirror International Publishers Limited
Printed by Grafos S. A. Arte sobre papel, Barcelona, Spain.
ISBN 0 7234 19183

For full details of all Times Mirror International Publishers Limited titles please write to Times Mirror International Publishers, Lynton House, 7–12 Tavistock Square, London, WC1H 9LB.

A CIP catalogue record for this book is available from the British Library.

Library of Congress Cataloging-in-Publication Data has been applied for.

Acknowledgements

The majority of the newly introduced illustrations derive from the author's own collection—as always, produced with the cooperation of his colleagues in the Oral Medicine Unit of the Liverpool University Dental Hospital (Mrs Anne Field, Ms Emma Varga and Mrs Janet Speechley). The illustrations in the section on HIV-associated lesions have been provided predominantly by Professor David Wray and Dr D. H. Felix of the Glasgow Dental Hospital and School, whose contributions are gratefully ackowledged.

Chapter 1

Infections of the Oral Mucosa

The normal mouth contains a wide range of bacterial and fungal organisms, many of which are potentially pathogenic. Control of these organisms is carried out by two main mechanisms: the local influence of the saliva, which contains a range of antibacterial substances (including IgA) and also exerts a protective washing and coating effect on the oral mucosa; and the integrity or otherwise of the individual's overall immune status, which is the overriding factor. If the immune status is compromised, previously commensal organisms may begin to behave in a pathogenic manner. The frequent occurrence of candidal infections of the oral mucosa in immunocompromised patients illustrates this, as *Candida* spp. are present in the mouths of a high proportion of normal individuals without producing any form of lesion.

Other oral infective conditions represent the first response of the patient to the infective agent, rather than a disturbance of a pre-existing host-commensal balance. The majority of oral viral infections are of this kind (**Table 1**).

TABLE 1

Type of Virus	Clinical manifestation
Herpes simplex (HSV)	Primary herpetic stomatitis Recurrent labial herpes Recurrent intraoral herpes
Herpes zoster virus (HZV)	Orofacial herpes zoster ('shingles')
Epstein–Barr virus (EBV)	Burkitt's lymphoma Infective mononucleosis ('glandular fever')
Coxsackie virus	Herpangina Hand-foot-mouth disease Pharyngitis
Papillomavirus (HPV)	Papillomas, warts Focal epithelial hyperplasia

Viral infections

Herpes simplex

Primary herpetic stomatitis

By far the most common acute viral infection seen in the oral cavity is primary herpetic stomatitis. This is the result of infection by the herpes simplex virus (HSV), also known as the herpes hominis virus (HHV). Until relatively recently, the great majority of oral herpetic infections have been due to the type 1 virus (HSV1), the type two virus (HSV2) being largely confined to lesions in the genital area. This distinction has now become less clear, and a significant proportion of oral infections are now found to be due to HSV2. This, however, has not been found to affect the clinical picture in any way—the lesions are indistinguishable.

Primary herpetic stomatitis results from the first infection by the virus, although the initial infection may be subclinical. It is most common in children and young adults, but may occur at any age. The lesions are initially vesicular (**1**), and may occur at any site in the oral cavity. Usually they are widespread. The vesicles quickly rupture, and it is unusual to see them intact. This breakdown results in the production of ulcerated areas covered by yellow sloughs (**2**). Malaise and pyrexia are usually present, particularly in children, and there is often marked cervical adenopathy.

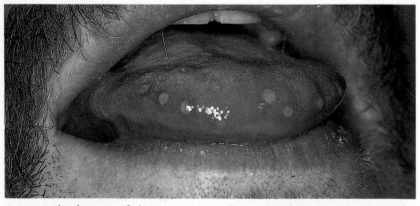

1 Vesicular lesions of the tongue in early primary herpetic stomatitis. The lesions have not, as yet, begun to break down—this vesicular stage is relatively transient.

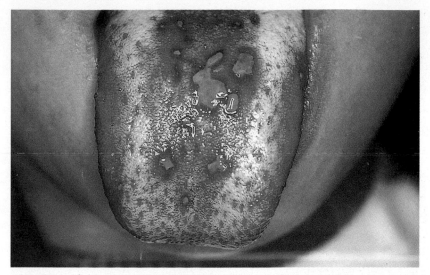

2 Lesions of the tongue in primary herpetic stomatitis at a slightly later stage than those shown in **1**. In this six-year-old patient, the lesions have partly broken down with the production of ulcerated areas covered by yellow sloughs.

In primary herpes, the majority of lesions are confined to the oral mucosa, although in some patients the lips and perioral mucosa may also be affected (**3** and **4**). In the later stages of acute herpetic stomatitis, secondary infection may play an important part in the creation of discomfort and in the extension of the lesions (**5** and **6**). Stagnation occurs, and the tongue may become heavily coated (**5**).

At this stage the patient is often in considerable pain, largely due to secondary bacterial infection. For this reason, antibacterial therapy (such as tetracycline mouthwashes), may give considerable relief, although the viral component of the infection is quite unaffected by the treatment. There may be a marked gingivitis (**7**), sometimes described by the term 'herpetic gingivostomatitis'. In children, the gingivitis (**8**) may look similar to that seen in some acute leukaemias, and a blood examination is often necessary to differentiate between these possibilities.

It should be stressed that primary herpetic stomatitis occurs only once in a healthy patient—an apparent recurrence indicates either a faulty diagnosis or an immunocompromised patient.

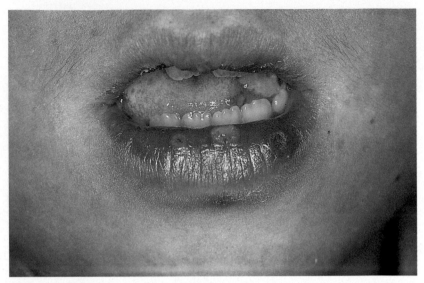

3 Lesions of the lips in primary herpetic stomatitis.

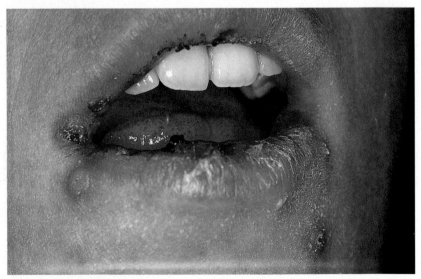

4 Vesicular lesions of the lips and perioral skin accompanying the intra-oral lesions in primary herpetic stomatitis.

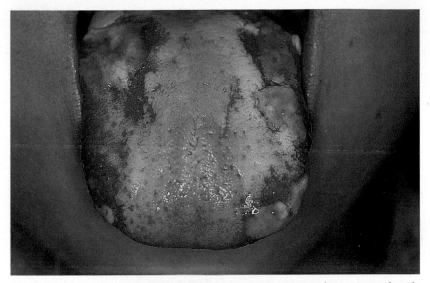

5 A later stage in primary herpetic stomatitis. Stagnation has occurred with the production of a heavily coated tongue.

6 The breakdown and spread of the initial lesions of primary herpetic stomatitis, with secondary infection occurring, is shown here. A few small vesicles are still present.

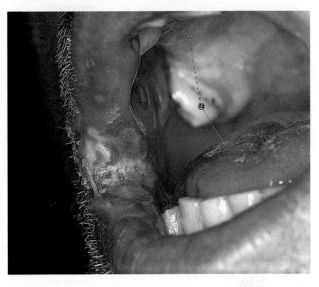

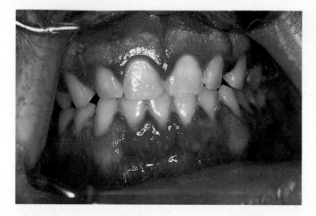

7 Gingivitis in primary herpetic stomatitis. There is a red marginal gingivitis contrasting with the white appearance of the rest of the gingivae caused by the retention of stagnation products.

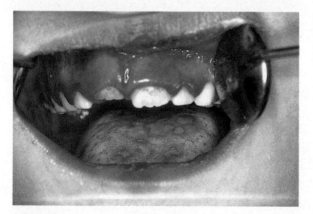

8 A rather proliferative gingivitis in a child with primary herpetic stomatitis.

Primary herpes simplex

•**Diagnosis:** Clinical, viral growth, rising antibody titres over ten days, electron microscopy. Epithelial smears show non-specific virus-induced changes.

•**Important differential diagnoses:** From erythema multiforme (see Chapter 7) and from acute leukaemia, especially in children (see Chapter 4).

Recurrent herpes simplex

An episode of primary herpetic infection stimulates a wide and variable range of immune responses, both cell-mediated and humoral. Viral material remains latent in the orofacial sensory nerves and, in about 50% of all patients, may become reactivated with the production of recurrent lesions, usually on or about the mucocutaneous junction of the lips. The recurrences are initially vesicular, but rapidly break down to form the familiar crusted lesions (cold sores) (**9** and **10**). These last for approximately ten days, then heal without scar formation. The recurrences may be precipitated by exposure to unaccustomed strong sunlight or by trauma, such as occurs in dental treatment.

Very occasionally, there is a recurrence of infection in intraoral sites, with the production of multiple small vesicles, usually on the gingivae (**11**). Recurrent intraoral HSV infections in an immunologically intact patient are practically always minor in nature, and are much less troublesome than the primary episode. In immunocompromised patients, orofacial herpetic infections may be severe and widespread, particularly in patients with AIDS or with blood dyscrasias (**12**).

9 Erythematous prevesicular lesions in recurrent facial herpes.

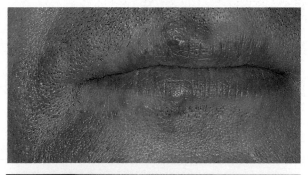

10 A typical single crusted lesion of recurrent facial herpes.

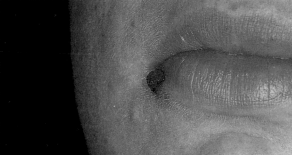

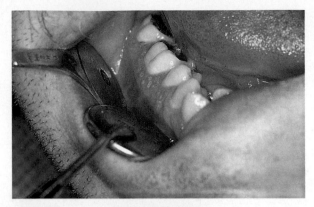

11 Recurrent intra-oral herpes. The small vesicular lesions on the gingivae are characteristic of this very rare condition. They are not particularly painful.

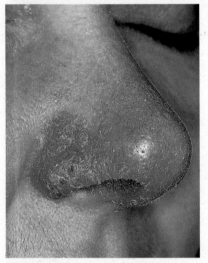

12 Recurrent facial herpes in a patient with chronic lymphocytic leukaemia.

Recurrent herpes simplex

•**Diagnosis:** Principally clinical, particularly dependent on history. Can be confirmed by epithelial smears or viral growth. Associated conditions are: the common cold, leukaemia, pneumonia and during immunosuppression. Precipitated by sunlight or trauma.

•**Important differential diagnosis:** From early carcinoma of lower lip, especially in older male patients. (See Chapter 10.)

Herpes zoster

Primary infection by the herpes zoster virus (HZV or HHV3) may cause chickenpox, although it may be subclinical and remain unnoticed. Reactivation of the virus, latent in sensory nerve fibres, may result in the production of recurrent lesions ('shingles'), which may be extremely painful and debilitating. The most common site is on the trunk, in which there is a distribution of a single dermatome, but branches of the trigeminal nerve or cervical nerves may be involved (**13** and **14**).

The lesion is initially a red, papular rash which rapidly becomes vesicular, the vesicles often being haemorrhagic. The ophthalmic division of the trigeminal nerve is often involved, and the eye may be badly affected. Intra-oral lesions—often unilateral—may also occur, closely resembling those in herpes simplex. Intra-oral lesions in herpes zoster infections rarely occur in the absence of skin lesions.

Perhaps the most distressing factor in herpes zoster is the possible development of post-herpetic neuralgia in the distribution of the affected nerve. This is a particularly intractable condition to treat. Occasionally, primary herpes simplex may simulate herpes zoster

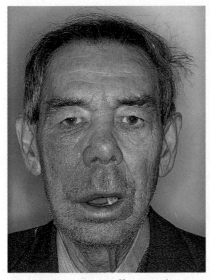

13 Herpes zoster affecting the second division of the right trigeminal nerve. The accurate anatomical distribution of the lesions is typical.

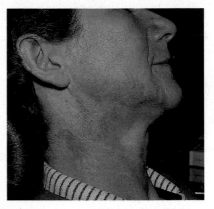

14 In this patient with a herpes zoster infection, the cervical nerves C2 and C3 were involved.

with a distribution which may be unilateral (**15**) or may be confined to the distribution of one branch of the trigeminal nerve. In these cases, differentiation between the two conditions may be dependent on the availability of sophisticated laboratory facilities.

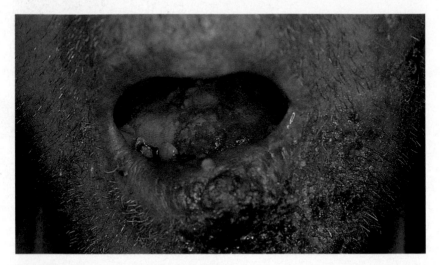

15 This severe primary herpes simplex infection gives the initial impression, because of its unilateral distribution, of herpes zoster.

Herpes zoster

Diagnosis: Clinical, viral growth, antibody studies, epithelial smears.

Epstein–Barr virus

The Epstein–Barr virus (EBV) is a form of herpes virus with numerous tentative disease associations. It is most clearly involved in the Burkitt lymphoma and in glandular fever (infective mononucleosis). Patients with glandular fever may have marked cervical lymphadenopathy, sore throats and tonsillitis, and, occasionally, quite severe oral ulceration (**16**). This, however, is non-specific, and is very unlikely to lead to a diagnosis of the generalised condition on its own account.

16 Palatal ulceration in infective mononucleosis (glandular fever).

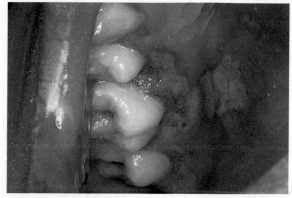

Epstein–Barr virus

Diagnosis: Infective mononucleosisis diagnosed by Paul–Bunnel test for heterophil antibodies, abnormal lymphocytes in blood.

Coxsackie viruses

Although herpetic infections are the most common viral diseases appearing in the oral medicine clinic, others are seen from time to time. Most of these, however, are relatively transient, and rarely present for diagnosis as oral medical problems. Probably the most common group of oropharyngeal viral infections are those associated with the Coxsackie group of viruses.

Herpangina (Coxsackie A group viruses) presents as a sore throat, self-limiting and lasting in total up to ten days. Initially, there may be a number of very ill-defined vesicles on the soft palate orpharynx (**17**) which may coalesce to form larger ulcers. Some Coxsackie infections (virus types A5, A10 and A16) may cause individual oral ulcers (**18**) and may be responsible for the condition known as hand–foot–mouth disease (not associated with foot and mouth disease in cattle). In this condition, oral bullae are accompanied by a vesicular rash on the hands and feet (**19** and **20**).

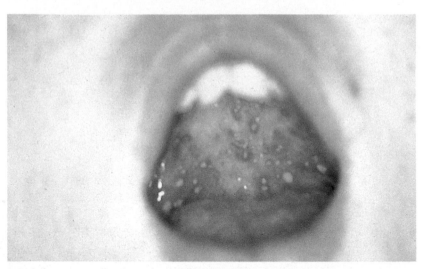

17 Herpangina—a pharyngitis caused in this case by the Coxsackie A4 virus. There is a diffuse erythema of the palate with some small transient vesicles.

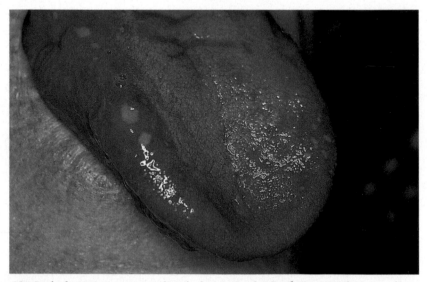

18 Oral ulceration associated with the Coxsackie A16 virus. In this case there was only oral ulceration present.

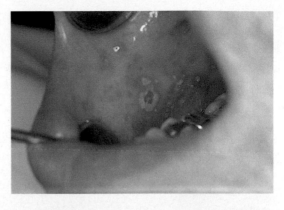

19 A ruptured oral bulla in hand-foot-mouth disease associated with the Coxsackie A16 virus. (See Figure **20**.)

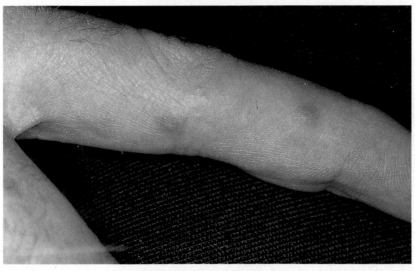

20 Vesicular lesions of the fingers in the patient shown in **19**. There were also lesions present on the feet.

Coxsackie virus infection

Diagnosis: Clinical, viral growth—rarely necessary because of mild and transient symptoms.

Papillomaviruses

Papillomaviruses (HPV) have been associated with a number of disease processes—particularly neoplasms, although a cause-and-effect relationship is often difficult to establish. The relationship with oral papillomas and verrucas is fairly well established (see Chapter 9 for a discussion of these lesions).

An interesting condition, which seems to be associated with the presence of a specific type of HPV, is focal epithelial hyperplasia (Heck's disease), although there is also thought to be a genetic factor involved. The patients in this self-limiting condition are largely children from coloured African, Eskimo and American Indian origin, although a few white European patients have been recorded. Multiple raised plaques appear on the buccal and labial mucosa, which retains its colour and texture (**21**). The histological changes in the epithelium seem strongly indicative of a viral involvement, and specific staining techniques seem to confirm the involvement of a HPV. The condition eventually regresses without treatment.

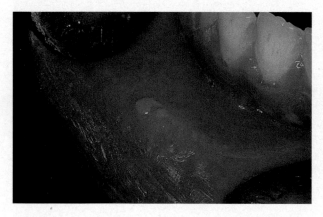

21 Lesions on the labial mucosa in focal epithelial hyperplasia (Heck's disease).

Papillomaviruses

Diagnosis: Clinical/histological. Virus can be identified in tissues by highly sophisticated immuno-histopathological techniques.

Candidal infections

Both 'candidiasis' and 'candidosis' are terms used to describe candidal infections, although microbiologists have recently adopted the term 'candidosis'. However, 'candidiasis' is more generally recognised and so will be used in the present context.

Candida spp.—largely, but not entirely, *Candida albicans*—may be found in the oral cavities of a high proportion of clinically normal individuals. The precise figures quoted depend entirely on the sampling methods used. This commensal–host relationship may be disturbed by any changes in the host —either local or systemic—which reduce the surveillance of the organisms. Clinical candidiasis is therefore a reflection of some degree of abnormality in the patient. This may range from an entirely local factor—such as the covering of the mucosa with a denture—to a profound, generalised disease process resulting in loss of immune competence.

The classification of the forms of oral candidiasis has been the subject of much debate—several variants on the groupings used here have been suggested, but these do not significantly alter the clinical implications of the classification (**Table 2**).

TABLE 2 Classification of Oral Candidiasis	
Type of candidiasis	**Alternative name**
Acute psedomembranous	Thrush
Chronic pseudomembranous	
Acute atrophic	Acute eythematous Antibiotic sore mouth
Chronic atrophic	Denture sore mouth Denture stomatitis
Chronic mucocutaneous	
Chronic hyperplastic	(*Candida* leukoplakia)
Angular cheilitis	

Median Rhomboid glossitis

Pseudomembranous candidiasis

Acute pseudomembranous candidiasis (thrush) is a common manifestation of oral candidiasis; the organisms are present on the surface of the mucous membrane as a network of hyphae, in which are enmeshed epithelial cells, bacteria and debris-forming white plaques on the surface (**22**). Some hyphae penetrate superficially into the epithelium, forming a loose attachment which is readily severed by wiping off the plaques, leaving a red and bleeding surface behind. This is a useful preliminary diagnostic test.

Thrush may be found in very young infants or very old individuals with apparently good health, but is otherwise a marker of some abnormality related to the lowering of body defences. It is very common in HIV-positive patients—75% develop thrush at some stage of their infection. It is thought that its appearance in the very young or very old is a marker of undeveloped or failing physiological responses in the absence of any definable disease process.

'Chronic pseudomembranous candidiasis' is a term recently introduced in recognition of the fact that, in some patients, pseudomembranous candidiasis is not necessarily an acute condition, but may be present over a long period of time (**23**). This form of candidiasis, although it is associated with generalised ill health, is without the multisystem involvement found in chronic mucocutaneous candidiasis.

Pseudomembraneous candidiasis

Diagnosis: Clinical, the 'wipe off' test. Laboratory diagnosis from direct smears, swabs and culture. Other sampling methods available, e.g. imprint cultures and rinsing techniques.

Associated conditions: A wide range of diseases leading to a lack of immune surveillance, including anaemias and related conditions, diabetes mellitus and HIV-related diseases (**49**).

Important differential diagnosis: From lichen planus or other intrinsic white patches of oral mucosa.

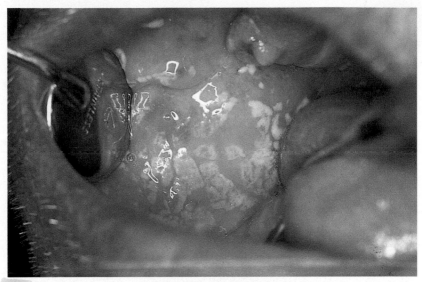

22 Acute pseudomembranous candidiasis ('thrush').

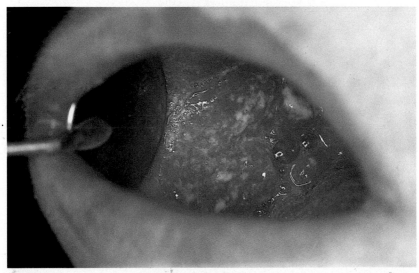

23 Chronic pseudomembranous candidiasis resulting from long-term candidal infection in a patient with myasthenia gravis.

Acute atrophic (erythematous) candidiasis

Acute atrophic (erythematous) candidiasis is often described as being like pseudomembranous candidiasis, but without the pseudomembrane. The epithelium is atrophic, contains embedded hyphae and readily breaks down to form painful erosions (**24**). It often affects the tongue—either as a marker of complex disease (**25**) or, more commonly, as a complication of antibiotic therapy. The term 'erythematous candidiasis' has recently come into more frequent use with the recognition of its characteristic appearance in HIV-positive patients (**50**). It is suggested that erythematous candidiasis represents a preliminary stage in the onset of pseudomembranous candidiasis in immunodeficient patients, but this has not, as yet, been confirmed.

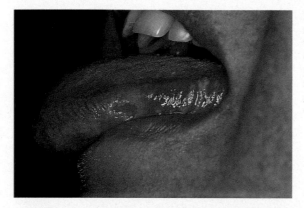

24 A patch of acute atrophic candidiasis on the left lateral margin of the tongue. The patient had an adrenal neoplasm leading to gross overproduction of corticosteroids.

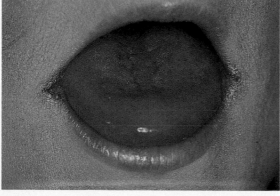

25 Atrophic candidiasis in a patient with a complex immune abnormality. This, although long-standing, shows the markers of acute candidiasis (including severe discomfort), and should probably be classified with other acute lesions.

Chronic atrophic candidiasis

Chronic atrophic candidiasis (denture sore mouth, denture stomatitis) is a very common manifestation of candidiasis. It results from the secondary infection of traumatised tissues below a dental appliance. In spite of its alternative description, it is quite painless. In the most common form (Newton's type 2) there is uniform erythema of the mucosa confined to the upper denture-bearing area (**26**). In type 1 there are punctate areas of erythema, representing localised atrophic changes (**27**), and in type 3 there is a nodular hyperplastic epithelial reaction to the long-lasting trauma, with some interspersed atrophic areas (**28**).

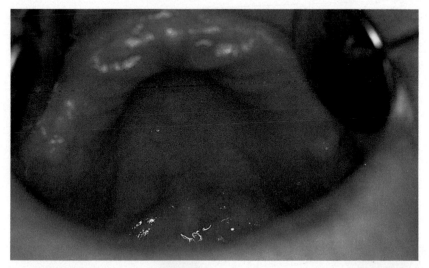

26 Chronic atrophic candidiasis (denture stomatitis, denture sore mouth) below a full upper denture. This (Newton's type 2) is the most common form.

25

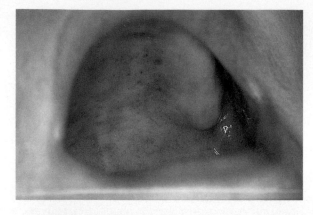

27 Chronic atrophic candidiasis type 1 with localised areas of atrophy on the denture-bearing area.

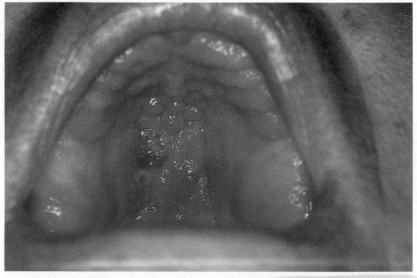

28 Chronic atrophic candidiasis type 3 with a papillary hyperplastic epithelial response and intermediate areas of atrophy.

Chronic atrophic candidiasis

Diagnosis: Predominantly clinical. *Candida* can be cultured from swabs taken from the palate or from the fitting surface of a denture.

Angular cheilitis

Angular cheilitis is a condition often associated with chronic atrophic candidiasis in denture wearers. This is particularly the case when the dentures are old and ill-fitting, or where alveolar re-absorption has led to deep folding at the angles of the mouth. In most patients, the area becomes heavily infected by *Candida*, which thrive in the environment of moist skin (**29**). However, not all lesions of angular cheilitis are infected by candida; some are infected by bacteria, usually staphylococci, either alone or in conjunction with *Candida* (**30**).

In long-standing cases of candidal angular cheilitis, granulomatous lesions containing organisms may form (**31**). These may be difficult to eradicate, except by surgical means. The relationship between angular cheilitis (and other candidal infections) and leukoplakia is demonstrated in Chapter 9. Angular cheilitis is a frequent oral manifestation of anaemias and related conditions (see Chapter 4)—a haematology screen should always be carried out if there is no evident cause for angular cheilitis.

Angular cheilitis

Diagnosis: Clinical. Swabs for laboratory growth to distinguish between candidal and staphylococcal infection. Haematology screening when indicated.

Important differential diagnosis: From angular lesions of oral Crohn's disease (see Chapter 5).

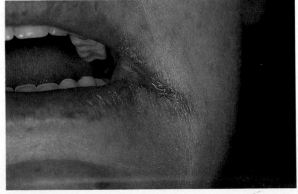

29 Candidal angular cheilitis associated with poorly fitting dentures and 'denture sore mouth'

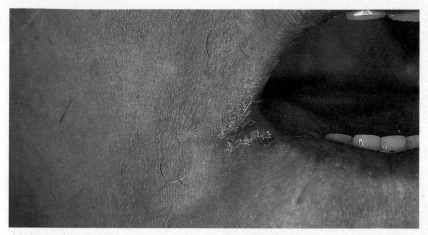

30 Angular cheilitis in which the infecting organism is not *Candida*, but *Staphylococcus aureus*.

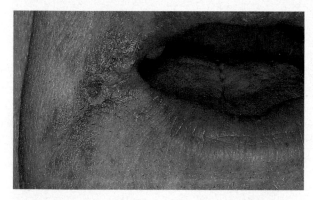

31 Granulomatous angular cheilitis following a long-standing candidal infection.

Chronic mucocutaneous candidiasis

The term 'chronic mucocutaneous candidiasis' (CMC) is used to describe a group of relatively rare conditions in which there are persistent candidal infections of the skin, mouth and nail beds (**32**, **33** and **34**). In some (but not all) patients, there is a clear genetic background to the condition, and in some cases there is also an associated autoimmune-endocrine disorder such as hypoparathyroidism or Addison's disease (the 'endocrine candidiasis syndrome'). In spite of much investigation, there remains a great deal of confusion about this group of conditions, and the precise immune defect involved is not easily identified. Management is very difficult in most cases.

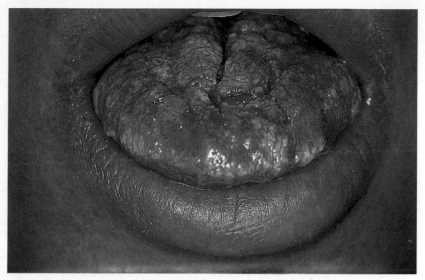

32 Chronic mucocutaneous candidiasis (CMC)—persistent oral candidiasis, associated in this patient with nailbed candidal infection (see **33**).

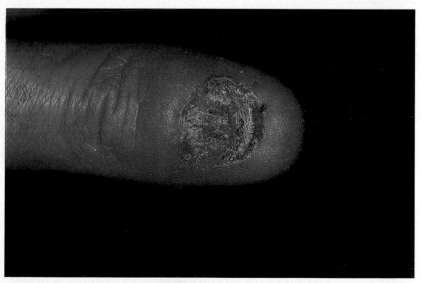

33 An infected fingernail of the patient with CMC shown in **32**.

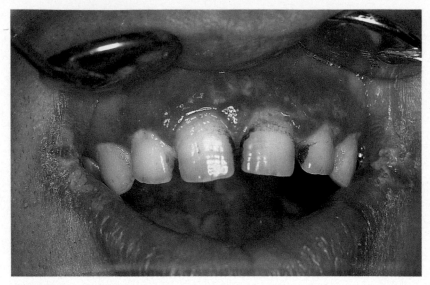

34 Diffuse candidal gingivitis in a patient with CMC—not the same patient as shown in **32** and **33**.

Chronic mucocutaneous candidiasis

Diagnosis: Cinical, with special emphasis on history and family-background. Complex endocrinological investigations may be necessary in endocrine-related cases.

Chronic hyperplastic candidiasis

'Chronic hyperplastic candidiasis' is a term synonymous with candidal leukoplakia. (This condition will be dealt with in Chapter 9, together with other leukoplakias.) A condition with a somewhat similar characteristic (e.g., the uncertain nature of the candidal involvement) is median glossitis (see Chapter 3).

Bacterial Infections

Primary bacterial infections of the oral mucosa in patients with an intact immune system are relatively unusual. In the patient with an impaired immune response (from whatever cause), they are more common although, even in these circumstances, viral and candidal infections are much more frequent.

Streptococcal stomatitis

Streptococcal stomatitis (or gingivo-stomatitis) has been long described as a true entity, and there is no doubt that streptococci may be cultured from some patients with a diffuse stomatitis and gingivitis (**35**). These patients often have an associated tonsilitis and pharyngitis, with mild systemic signs of toxaemia. However, it is debatable whether this condition represents a primary bacterial infection or secondary infection following a primary viral stomatitis. Staphylococcal angular cheilitis has already been described (**30**).

35

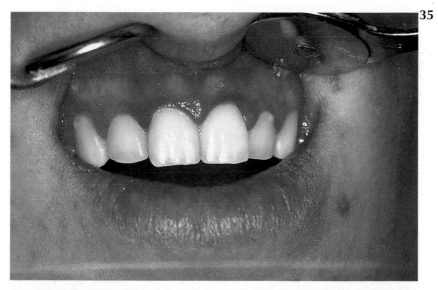

35 'Streptococcal gingivostomatitis'. This is the clinical picture in this condition of uncertain aetiology—a generalised stomatitis with shiny red gingivae.

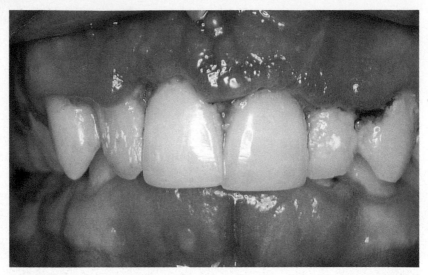

36 Acute ulcerative gingivitis in a relatively early stage. The typical loss of the papillae is already evident.

Acute ulcerative gingivitis

Acute ulcerative gingivitis (AUG) or necrotising ulcerative gingivitis, (NUG) is a common condition with a rather uncertain aetiology. There is always an associated overgrowth of Vincent's organisms (*Borrelia vincentii* and *Fusiformis fusiformis*) in the affected areas, but there is evidence that a simple infection by these organisms is not the cause of the disease. However, on a practical basis, elimination of these organisms coincides with clinical remission of symptoms. In this condition there is tenderness and bleeding of the gingivae, with ulceration initially and predominantly affecting the interdental papillae (**36**). As the condition progresses, there is lateral spread of the ulceration to affect the gingival margins (**37**). There may be malaise, lymphadenitis, pyrexia and marked halitosis. Eventual resolution may take place with some damage to the gingival contour. Most patients with AUG are otherwise healthy young adults, but it may also occur as an opportunist infection in the face of lowered resistance, either local or generalised. It may occur secondarily in patients with oral viral infections (**38**), and will be later mentioned as an important oral HIV-associated lesion. Its aggressive spread to form the highly destructive lesions of cancrum oris is also illustrated and commented upon in **48**.

37 Acute ulcerative gingivitis in a more advanced stage. Lateral spread along the gingival margins is occurring.

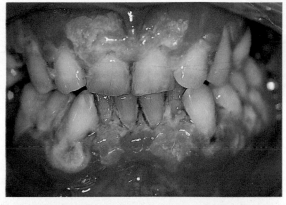

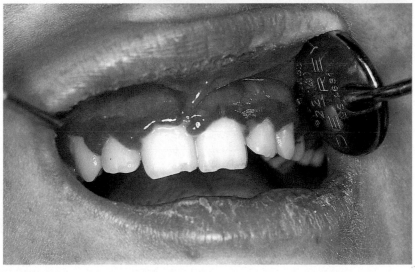

38 Acute ulcerative gingivitis occurring secondary to acute herpetic stomatitis.

Acute ulcerative gingivitis

Diagnosis: Clinical. Laboratory diagnosis by direct smears taken from lesions—culture of organisms very difficult.

Associated conditions: Leukaemias, HIV infection, other debilitating conditions.

Syphilis

The oral primary syphilitic lesion (chancre) most commonly appears on the lip (**39**), less frequently on the tongue (**40**). It develops some 2–3 weeks after infection as an indurated swelling with a red glazed surface. This later becomes crusted on the lip (**39**). These lesions are moderately painful, and the patient may at this stage develop enlarged and palpable regional lymph nodes.

The primary lesions are highly infectious, the surface fluid containing large numbers of *Treponema pallidum*, and they last from 1–5 weeks. Secondary stage lesions have in the past been described as mucous patches with a characteristic appearance, but it is now accepted that many secondary syphilitic lesions may appear as relatively non-specific ulcers (**41**).

The secondary stage is generally described as starting approximately six weeks after infection. Some patients, such as the patient shown in **39**, develop secondary oral lesions whilst the primary lesion is still present. Secondary lesions heal without trace after 2–6 weeks.

Tertiary syphilis may appear in the oral cavity in two ways: gumma formation, most commonly in the palate, which may cause bone loss and soft tissue distortion (**42**) and may lead to palatal perforation (**43**); or the formation of tertiary lesions of chronic glossitis with overlying leukoplakia. This is now a relative rarity, although in the past syphilis was considered to be one of the most significant factors in the aetiology of leukoplakia. This condition is illustrated in Chapter 9. The dental markers of congenital syphilis are shown in Chapter 12.

Syphilis

Diagnosis: In primary and secondary lesions: direct dark ground microscopy of material from surface of lesion. Fluorescent treponaemal antibody test (FTA), positive 90% in primary stage. Venereal disease research laboratory test (VDRL), positive 75% in primary stage. Both tests approach 100% in secondary stage.

Associated diseases: Other sexually transmitted diseases.

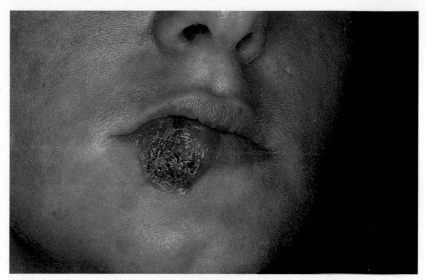

39 Primary syphilitic lesion (chancre) on lower lip.

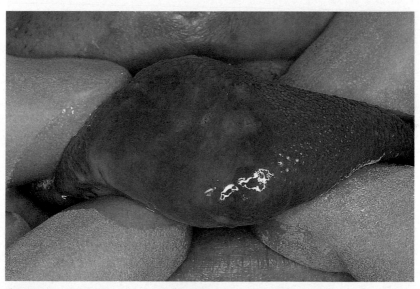

40 Primary syphilitic lesion of the tongue.

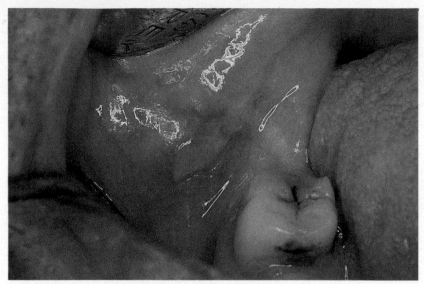

41 A secondary stage syphilitic ulcer of the buccal mucosa.

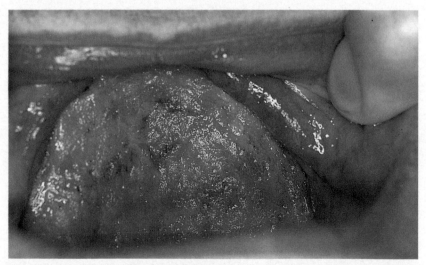

42 Tertiary syphilis—gumma formation in the palatal mucosa has led to distortion of the tissues. Although not evident in the illustration, there was also marked loss of palatal bone, with the formation of a small oro-nasal fistula.

43 A gumma has led to a large palatal defect in this very elderly patient. The disease had presumably remained latent for many years.

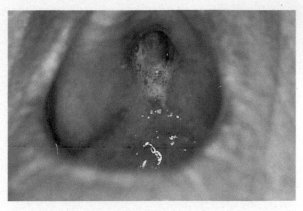

Tuberculosis

The classic appearance of oral tuberculosis as described in the recent past was of an ulcer secondary to uncontrolled pulmonary tuberculosis (**44**). This has now become very uncommon—at least in European conditions—but there are increasing indications that tuberculosis may be currently emerging as a significant cause of oral lesions with no clinically identifiable characteristic features. The lesion shown in **45** presented as a faint white patch with no clinical indication of its true nature as a tubercular lesion. Many other 'atypical' oral lesions have been described, and with the emergence of tuberculosis as an important sequel of the immunosupression associated with HIV infection, it may well be that oral tuberculosis may again become a more common condition. The development of drug-resistant strains of *M. tuberculosis* may be of great importance in this context.

Tuberculosis

Diagnosis: Initially histological (acid-fast organisms rarely seen in oral lesions). Culture and guinea-pig inoculation of material from fresh biopsy.

Associated diseases: Debilitating diseases, malnutrition, increasingly HIV-associated.

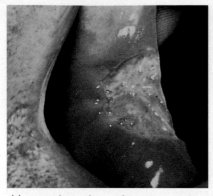 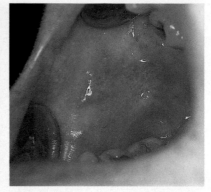

44 A tuberculous ulcer in a patient with active pulmonary tuberculosis.

45 Tuberculosis—this painless faint white patch on the buccal mucosa was found to have a tuberculoid histology on biopsy, and *M. tuberculosis* was incubated from the biopsy tissue. No other tubercular lesions were found in the patient.

Immunodeficiency

Immunodeficiencies may be classified as primary and secondary. Primary immunodeficiencies are relatively rare—in these patients, there is an intrinsic failure in the development of the immune system—usually genetically determined. Chronic mucocutaneous candidiasis, discussed and illustrated previously (**32**, **33** and **34**) is the most likely condition of this type to present with oral manifestations.

Secondary immunodeficiencies are not genetically determined and represent an adverse response of the immune system to some extrinsic factor. There are many such possible causes of secondary immunodeficiency (summarised in **Table 3**), the most significant until recently being the unwanted side effects of steroids, cytotoxic drugs and other immunosupressive agents used therapeutically. More recently, however, the spread of the HIV-induced Acquired Immunodeficiency Syndrome (AIDS) has become a dominant consideration. In patients with immune deficiencies of varying origins and degrees of severity, oral candidiasis is often an early and persistent marker of the condition.

A wide range of generalised diseases may be associated with secondary immunodeficiency. Diabetes mellitus, particularly when poorly controlled, often results in oral candidiasis, as do other endocrine disorders (**24**). A similar situation has been shown previously in a patient with myasthenia gravis (**23**). Immune deficiency is common in malignant disease—particularly in the leukaemias and lymphomas. Consequential oral infections of many kinds may occur—candidiasis and oro-facial herpes being the most common (see Figure **11**).

Iatrogenic (drug-induced) immunosupression is perhaps most commonly met as a complication of steroid therapy, either systemic or local. By far the most common oral manifestation is of candidiasis in some form (**46**). Steroid aerosols, used in the treatment of asthma, are a common cause of oro pharyngeal candidiasis. Aggressive immunosupressive therapy, as used (for example) in transplant procedures, is commonly followed by severe oral infections. The use of massive doses of steroids, often together with cytotoxic drugs, to prevent graft rejection may lead to extensive oral infections, not only by *Candida* spp., but also by a range of organisms which might, in the normal patient, be considered as commensal (**47**).

Malnutrition, either generalised or due to a specific deficiency state, may result in immunodeficiency and consequent oral changes. An extreme example of this is in cancrum oris—a condition most commonly now seen in children in some African countries. This condition

TABLE 3   Some Examples of Secondary Immunodeficiency

Disorder	Example	Oral manifestation*
Endocrine disease	Diabetes mellitus	Candidiasis (see **24**)
Autoimmune disease	Myasthenia gravis	Candidiasis (see **23**)
Malignancy	Leukaemias	Herpes zoster or simplex (see **12**)
Iatrogenic	Steroid therapy	Candidiasis (see **46**)
Malnutrition	Protein deficiency	Cancrum oris (see **48**)
Viral infection	HIV	Multiple (See **Tables 4** and **5**)

* These are examples only—more than one oral lesion may occur in some conditions, particularly in HIV infections.

represents a rapid spread of infection by the Vincent's organisms from a relatively localised site in the gingivae, which causes massive soft tissue destruction of the face (**48**). In the affected patients, there is a combination of pre-existing gross malnutrition and a viral infection—usually measles—which together cause a sufficient depression of the immune control mechanisms to allow the infection to spread aggressively. A similar condition may occur in some terminal leukaemic patients.

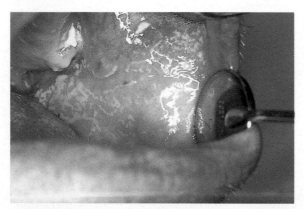

46 Acute membranous candidiasis (thrush) in a patient taking sytstemic steroids.

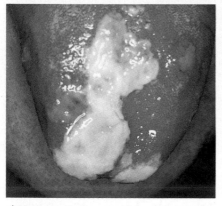

47 A staphylococcal lesion on the tongue of a patient undergoing intensive immunosuppressive therapy for rejection of a renal transplant.

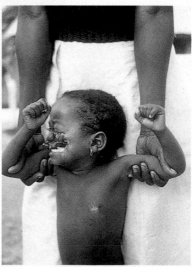

48 The results of cancrum oris in a Nigerian child.

HIV-associated lesions

A number of viral infections may result in secondary immune deficiencies of varying degrees of significance—for example, the role of measles in the aetiology of cancrum oris has been mentioned above. However, the current predominating interest in this field lies in the oral effects of the HIV and the profound immunosupression which may occur in infected patients. Oral lesions are often among the first indications of HIV infection, and are found in the majority of patients with fully developed AIDS. A wide range of possible oral manifestations of HIV infection have been recorded, but the currently widely accepted group of lesions strongly associated with HIV infection is shown in **Table 4**. Apart from these oral changes, cervical lymph node enlargement is also an important feature of all stages of HIV-associated disease.

TABLE 4 Oral Lesions with Strong HIV Association

Candidiasis

> Pseudomembranous
> Atrophic (erythematous)
> Hyperplastic
> Angular cheilitis

Hairy leukoplakia

Gingvival changes (HIV-specific)

> HIV gingivitis
> HIV periodontitis

Acute ulcerative gingivitis

Neoplasms

> Kaposi's sarcoma
> Lymphoma (non-Hodgkin's)

Candidal infections

Candidal infections are probably the most common oral manifestation of HIV infection at all stages. Often they are the first indication of the condition and it has been suggested that the unexplained onset of oral candidiasis in a patient in an at-risk group should be considered as being highly suggestive of HIV infection. Pseudo-membranous candidiasis (thrush) is the most common form, and is reported as being seen in 75% of HIV-positive patients (**49**). Atrophic (erythematous) candidiasis is also relatively common (**50**), and any of the other forms of candidiasis described above may occur.

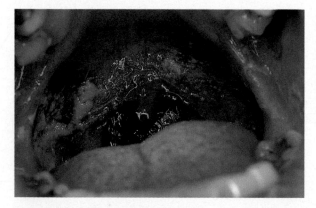

49 Pseudomembranous candidiasis on the palate of a HIV-infected patient. This patient also had an area of hyperplastic candidiasis on the buccal mucosa.

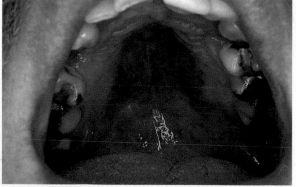

50 Erythematous candidiasis on the palate of a HIV-positive patient.

Hairy leukoplakia

Hairy leukoplakia is an idiosyncratic lesion which is said to be an invariable marker of HIV infection. It is described as a white, corrugated lesion on the lateral margin of the tongue (**51**), sometimes spreading to the ventral surface, which cannot be removed by rubbing. A few similar lesions have been described in other sites. Initially, this lesion was described as a form of candidal leukoplakia, but it is now thought that the Epstein–Barr virus is probably implicated in the aetiology, although this is not fully confirmed. A clinical diagnosis of hairy leukoplakia on appearance alone may be misleading—**52** shows thrush affecting the lateral margin of the tongue with a very similar appearance.

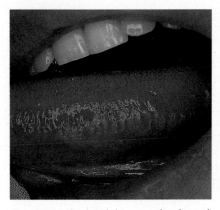 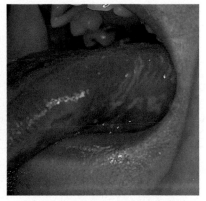

51 Hairy leukoplakia on the lateral margin of the tongue.

52 This is not a hairy leukoplakia, but a lesion of thrush which closely resembles it.

Periodontal changes

Periodontal changes have also been described in HIV-infected patients, ranging from a relatively mild gingivitis to a severe and rapidly progressive periodontitis (**53**), which may lead to loss of tooth attachment and of supporting bone. In some cases (necrotising gingivitis), the loss of bone and soft tissue may be extreme. Acute ulcerative gingivitis occurring in HIV-positive patients is similar to that seen in HIV-negative patients, but may be unusually severe and widespread.

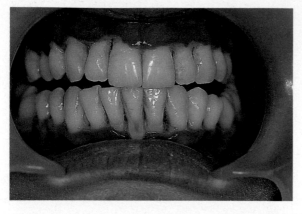

53 Severe HIV-associated periodontal disease.

Oral neoplasms

Various oral neoplasms have been described as occurring in HIV positive patients, but by far the most common is Kaposi's sarcoma. It may occur as an early oral manifestation of the infection, appearing in its first stages as a mucosal discolouration, most commonly on the hard palate (**54**). The behaviour of Kaposi's sarcoma appearing in HIV-positive patients may be much more aggressive than in HIV-negative patients; these aggressive lesions often affect the gingivae (**55**). Non-Hodgkin's lymphomas are the second most common oral malignant lesions seen in seropositive patients and, although controllable in general, may in some cases behave in a highly aggressive manner (**56** and **57**).

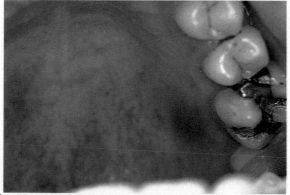

54 Early Kaposi's sarcoma on the hard palate.

55 Advanced Kaposi's sarcoma affecting the gingivae.

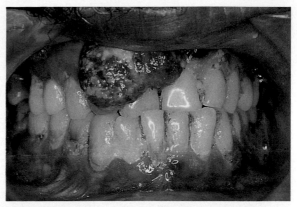

Lesions less strongly associated with HIV

Of the lesions currently classified as having less strong HIV connections (**Table 5**), viral infections—in particular, herpes simplex and herpes zoster infections—are the most frequent. Many would consider them to be classifiable among the conditions with 'strong connections'.

TABLE 5 **Oral Lesions with Less-Strong HIV Association**

Ulceration
    (Oral or pharyngeal)

Infections
    Viral*
    Bacterial
    Fungal (non-candidal)

Salivary gland swelling
    Xerostomia

Many other possible associations

---

* *Although not included in the currently accepted classification as a "strong association", herpes simplex and herpes zoster infections are frequently described in HIV-infected patients.*

45

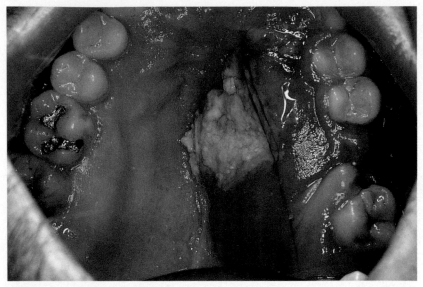

56 Non-Hodgkin's lymphoma affecting the hard palate in a HIV-infected patient.

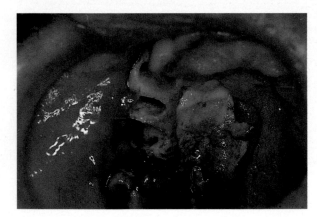

57 A more advanced stage of the lymphoma shown in **56** showing widespread tissue destruction.

Chapter 2

Recurrent Oral Ulceration

Recurrent oral ulceration (ROU, or recurrent aphthous ulceration [RAU], recurrent aphthae, recurrent aphthous stomatitis [RAS]) is a common condition. It has been suggested that some 20% of the European population may be affected at some time in their lives. There are a number of systemic diseases and diseases of the skin in which oral ulceration may occur or recur, but these are excluded from the group of conditions generally described as ROU. The generally accepted classification of ROU is the following three types:
- Minor aphthous ulceration;
- Major aphthous ulceration; and
- Herpetiform ulceration.

This classification is based almost entirely on the clinical features in each case. There may be some instances in which these are borderline or in which two types of ulceration may appear in the same patient. In spite of much effort, there is no clear understanding of the aetiology of any of these groups, but minor and major aphthous ulceration have some characteristics of autoimmune disease.

Herpetiform ulceration seems not to have these characteristics, and the aetiology remains unknown.

Minor aphthous ulceration

Minor aphthous ulceration (MiAU) is the most common form of ROU —80% of patients have this type. It may occur at any age, and is not rare in very young children. The incidence is approximately equally divided between the sexes. The ulcers are relatively small and appear in batches, typically of one to five, and most commonly on the buccal and labial mucosa (**58**). The tongue is sometimes affected, and occasionally the gingivae, but the ulceration very rarely extends to the palate or the pharynx. When occurring in the depths of a sulcus, the shape of the ulcers is modified and elongated (**59**).

After being present for a variable period (which, however, is predictable by each individual patient), the ulcers heal without scar formation. There is then a variable ulcer-free period before recurrence. In some patients, this a relatively regular pattern—ten days of ulceration followed by a three-week free period is common. In some patients there is no clear cyclic pattern, but a few experience continuous ulceration without a defined ulcer-free period. The site of ulceration may be selected by some form of trauma, especially in younger patients—the lower lip is often involved (**60** and **61**). The resulting ulcer is quite different from a simple traumatic ulcer (**62**).

In a few female patients the ulceration appears to be directly related to the menstrual cycle—the onset of ulceration is usually three days or so before the start of the menstrual period. Generally, MiAU is not related to any other disease process, but in some cases there is an association with haematological deficiencies. As an example, **63** illustrates a patient with problems of malabsorption, leading to moderately depressed serum folate and vitamin B12 levels. The ulceration, which had all the characteristics of typical RAU, ceased following treatment of the malabsorption and restoration of the deficient factors.

There is also a clear association between ROU of all types and coeliac disease (see Chapter 5). Many other generalised diseases are associated with non-specific oral ulceration, which is often wrongly described as 'aphthous' in the absence of the characteristics of any of the forms of ROU. A few patients develop genital ulcers of a kind similar to the oral ulcers; this is more common in patients with major aphthous ulcers.

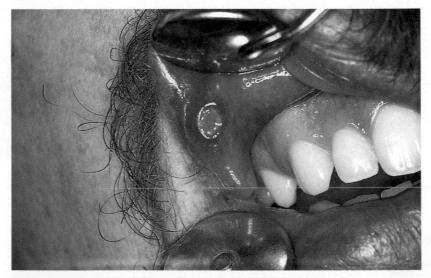

58 A typical minor aphthous ulcer on the labial mucosa.

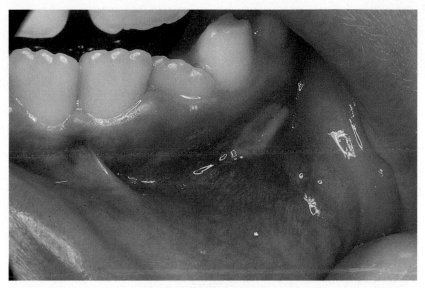

59 The elongated form of a minor aphthous ulcer when occurring deep in a sulcus.

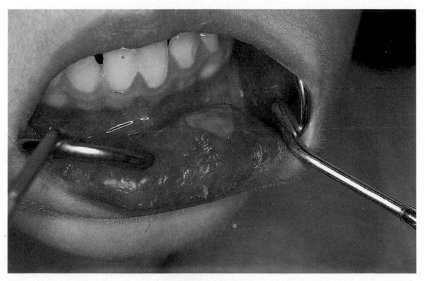

60 A traumatically precipitated aphthous ulcer on the lower lip of a child—see **61**. Also compare with **62**.

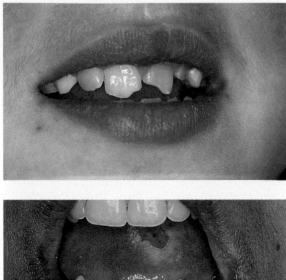

61 A fractured incisor causing mild trauma to the lower lip and stimulating production of the aphthous ulcer shown in **60**.

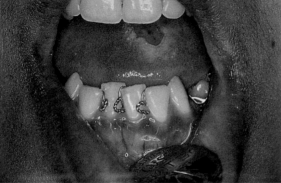

62 A typical true traumatic ulcer on the tongue, caused by irritation from orthodontic wiring. The white keratotic margin is characteristic of traumatic ulcers.

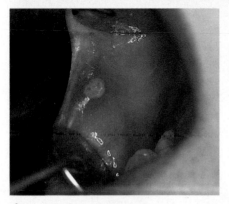

63 Aphthous ulceration associated with lowered folate and B12 levels due to malabsorption.

Minor apthous ulceration

Diagnosis: Clinical (see **Table 6**). Haematology screen to eliminate systemic background including coeliac disease.

Associated conditions: Genital ulceration, coeliac disease, anaemias, nutritional disturbances and Bechet's syndrome—see pp. 57–58.

Major aphthous ulceration

Major aphthous ulcers (MjAU) differ from the minor variety in their size—they are generally larger (**64**), sometimes very much so—but even more significantly in their duration. These ulcers may last for up to several months in some instances, and may heal with considerable scar formation (**65**). The commissures are often affected in this way (**66**). The oropharynx and soft palate are also often involved (**67**), with resultant tissue distortion and destruction if treatment is not successful (**68**). Most patients have no discernible cyclic pattern to their ulceration—it may run a completely unpredictable course, sometimes with periods of remission, sometimes with continuous episodes of ulcers. A proportion of patients give a history of MiAU—perhaps for some years—which then gradually progresses towards the major type. Orogenital ulceration is fairly often seen in patients with MjAU; the genital ulcers resemble the oral ulcers in their behaviour.

Major aphthous ulceration

Diagnosis: Clinical (see **Table 6**) and haematology screen.

Associated conditions: Genital ulceration, coeliac disease, anaemias, nutritional disturbances, Behçet's syndrome—see pages 57–58.

Important differential diagnosis: From carcinoma.

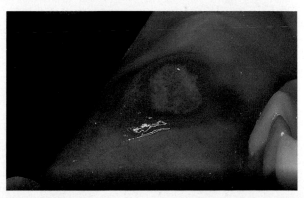

64 Major aphthous ulcer of lower lip.

TABLE 6 Recurrent Oral Ulceration

Diagnostic Features

Minor Aphthous Ulceration (MiAU)

>1–6 ulcers at a time
>Size small but variable—usually 2–10 mm
>Duration short—usually 10 days
>Usually cyclic
>Free period usually 3–4 weeks
>Site—mucosa excluding palate and oro-pharynx
>Heal without scars
>Occasional genital involvement

Major Aphthous Ulceration (MjAU)

>Usually 1 or 2 ulcers at a time
>Size prodominantly large—10 mm+
>Duration long—may be months
>Usually intermittent and non-cyclic
>Free period variable or none
>Site—all mucosa, including palate
>   and oro-pharynx
>Heal with scars
>More common genital involvement

Herpetiform Ulceration (HU)

>Many ulcers at a time
>Size small—under 2mm
>Duration variable—usually 1–2 weeks
>Non-cyclic
>Site—margins and tip of tongue, floor of mouth
>Heal without scars
>Genital involvement rare

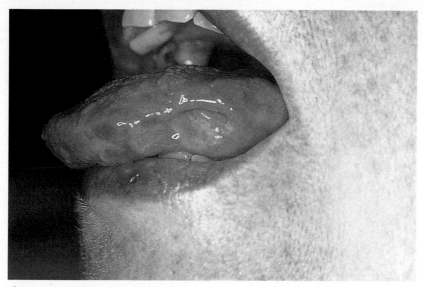

65 Scar on lateral margin of tongue of patient with major aphthous ulcers.

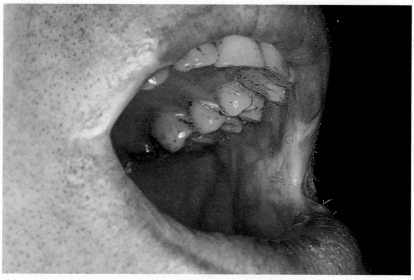

66 Commissural scarring in major aphthous ulceration.

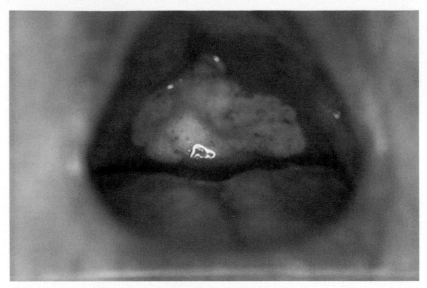

67 A large major aphthous ulcer of the soft palate.

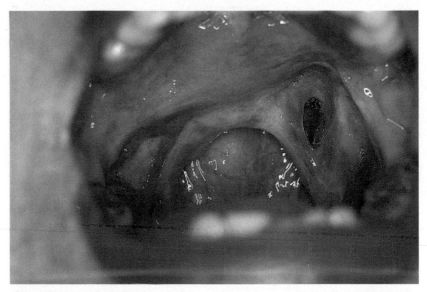

68 Tissue loss and distortion of the soft palate as a result of repeated major aphthous ulceration.

Herpetiform ulceration

Herpetiform ulceration (HU) is a relatively less common form of oral ulceration than either MiAU or MjAU. In spite of its name, herpetiform ulceration is not the result of infection by a herpes virus—the nomenclature originally reflected a suggested similarity to the skin disease dermatitis herpetiformis. In this form of ROU, the ulcers are small (in the order of 1 mm) and ill-defined, but often very painful (**69**). Sometimes several ulcers coalesce to form a single larger ulcer—but even these rarely exceed 2 mm or so in diameter. The site is characteristically in the anterior part of the mouth—the tip and lateral margins of the tongue, the floor of the mouth and, less frequently, the lips. There are usually many ulcers present in an attack, perhaps as many as fifty or one hundred (**70**). The duration of an attack is variable and unpredictable; these ulcers rarely have a cyclic pattern similar to that of MiAU, and usually heal without scar formation after some 7–14 days. Most patients are female (female : male = 2.6 : 1) and the 20–29 year age group is the most affected.

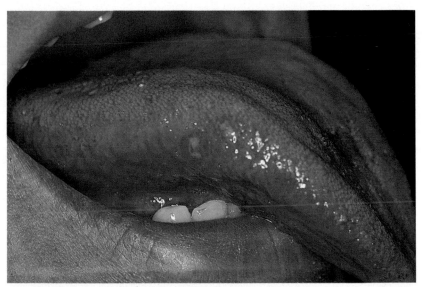

69 A solitary herpetiform ulcer on the lateral margin of the tongue.

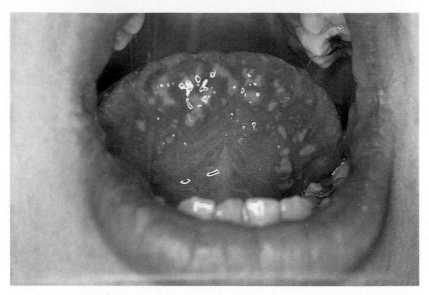

70 The usual pattern of herpetiform ulceration—many ulcers on the tip and lateral margins of the tongue.

Herpetiform ulceration

Diagnosis: Clinical (see **Table 6**), haematology screen.

Associated conditions: Coeliac disease, anaemias, nutritional disturbances and, rarely, genital ulceration.

Important differential diagnosis: From viral infections.

Behçet's syndrome

Behçet's syndrome is a multi-system disease of unknown aetiology, in which ROU (usually of the MjAU type) is a constant feature.

Other main components of the syndrome are genital ulceration and a variety of inflammatory and degenerative eye lesions. Other structures may also be involved in the disease, and are shown in **Table 7**. The patients are predominantly male (male : female = 2.3 : 1), and the onset of the disease is usually experienced in the third decade. There is a strong geographic bias, as a high proportion of patients are seen in Japan and Turkey, but some patients are seen in all parts of the world. This is a severely debilitating and potentially fatal condition of which the first manifestation may well be apparently uncomplicated ROU. **71** shows a patient with oral and genital ulceration, uveitis, skin lesions and mild arthitic changes who has maintained reasonable health for over 25 years—a very unusual situation. The chances of severe and disabling disease supervening in such circumstances are very high.

TABLE 7 Behçet's Syndrome

Clinical Features

Common manifestations (over 90% of patients)

> Recurrent oral ulceration
>> (MiAU, MjAU or HU)
>
> Genital ulceration
> Eye lesions (uveitis)

Less common manifestations

> Skin rashes and pustules
> Arthritis of major joints
> Vasculitis and thrombosis
> Neurological lesions—diffuse and
>> intracranial
>
> Haematuria
> Abdominal discomfort

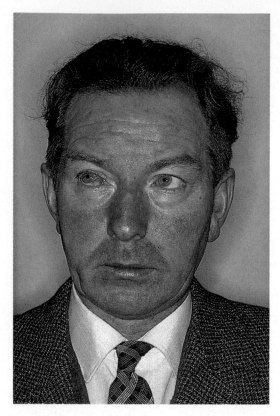

71 A patient with Behçet's syndrome, showing an erythematous skin rash and uveitis in the right eye.

Behçet's syndrome

Diagnosis: Main criteria: ROU, genital ulceration, uveitis. Conditions in **Table 7** support diagnosis. Specialist examination and diagnosis of each presenting condition is essential.

Important differential diagnosis: (In early stages) from skin diseases with oral and genital lesions (see Chapter 7).

Chapter 3

The Tongue and Lips

Although many of the conditions illustrated in this atlas involve the tongue together with other areas of the oral mucosa, there are a number of conditions which specifically involve the tongue alone. These are largely dependent on the specialised nature of the tongue epithelium and, in particular, on the behaviour of the papillae—in particular, the filliform papillae—which may undergo changes in their structure and distribution. The lips do not have such a specialised structure. However, being intermediate in site between the mucous membrane of the mouth and the skin of the face, lesions which might affect either may also affect the lips and the perioral area. In addition, there are a few lesions which have no parallels elsewhere and affect the lips only.

The Tongue

Significant developmental abnormalities of the tongue are very rare, unless minor variations in fissure pattern and size are included. Akyloglossia (tongue-tie) is the most common, and may be associated (as in the 13-year-old patient shown in **72** and **73**) with mild microglossia. Microglossia is almost invariably an isolated developmental abnormality—macroglossia, however, may occur in a variety of systemic conditions (see Chapter 11). Atrophic changes in the tongue may occur in some neurological diseases—as, for instance, in the hemiatrophy resulting from a lesion of the hypoglossal nerve (**74**).

Deep fissuring of the tongue is quite normal in some patients. It may not always be evident, however, and **75** and **76** demonstrate how fissures may become well marked or almost invisible according to the degree of lateral extension of the tongue. Although these deep, narrow fissures are of themselves symptomless, they may act as a site for stasis, infection and hence superficial irritation. It is often the case that conditions which cause tongue irritation are first felt predominantly in the fissures. However, only after the tongue has been affected by protracted inflammatory or degenerative conditions does the pattern of fissuring significantly change and become more marked (**77**). There are a number of normal variations in tongue morphology, involving slightly atypical fissure patterns which are well recognised and which have no relation to any abnormality (**78**, **79**). An uncommon condition in which a specific abnormal tongue fissure pattern is involved is the mysterious Melkersson–Rosenthal syndrome (see Chapter 6).

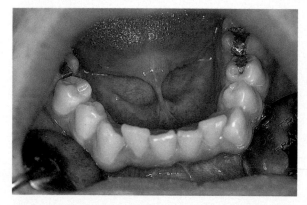

72 Ankyloglossia (tongue tie) in a 13-year-old patient—a relatively common, minor developmental abnormality.

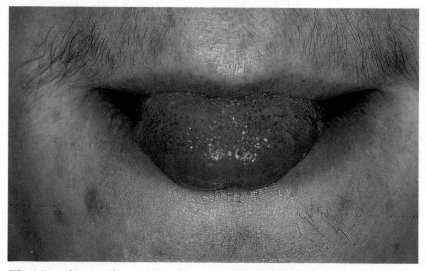

73 Microglossia. The patient's tongue is fully extended This is the same patient seen in **72**. The tongue tie is largely responsible for the inability to protrude.

74 Left-sided hemiatrophy of the tongue resulting from a lower motor neurone lesion affecting the hypoglossal nerve.

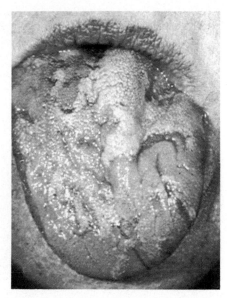

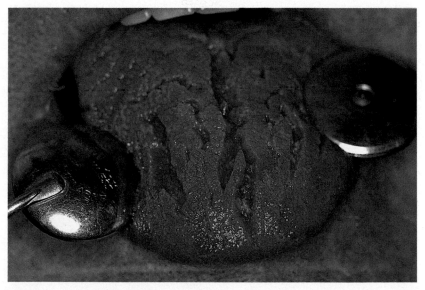

75 Deep tongue fissures shown up by lateral spreading of the tongue.

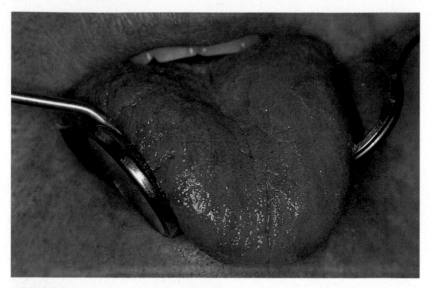

76 When the tongue is laterally compressed, rather than extended, the fissures seen in **75** are almost invisible.

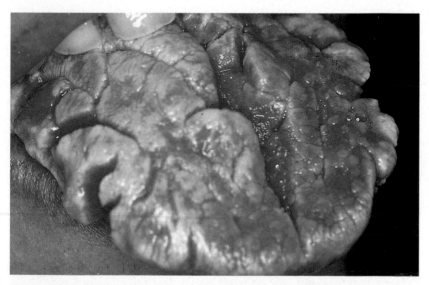

77 Exaggerated fissuring of the tongue as a result of long-term infection in chronic mucocutaneous candidiasis.

78 A slightly unusual but quite normal pattern of tongue morphology, known as 'crenated tongue.'

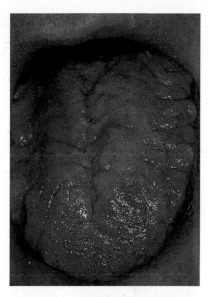

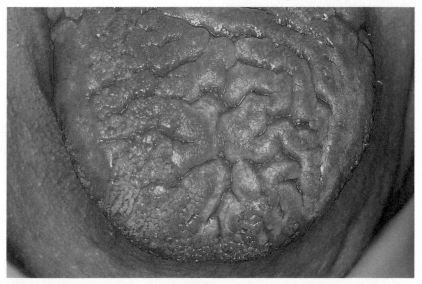

79 The so-called 'scrotal tongue'—again, a normal variant.

Hairy tongue

Hairy tongue (**80, 81**) is brought about by elongation of the filliform papillae and is of unknown aetiology, although a number of precipitating factors are recognised. Many cases follow a course of antibiotic therapy—either systemic or local—but others are apparently entirely idiopathic. The black or brown colouration of the elongated papillae is of unknown origin; it is usual to ascribe these colours to the presence of pigment-forming bacteria, but this in fact cannot be demonstrated.

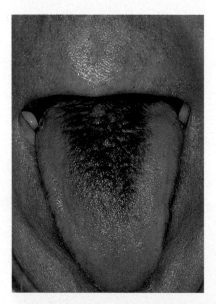

80 Black hairy tongue with no known precipitating factor.

Hairy tongue

Diagnosis: Clinical.

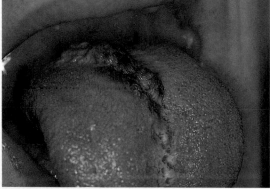

81 Brown hairy tongue restricted to the area bordering a deep midline fissure.

Depapillation

Partial depapillation of the tongue, particularly at the tip, may occur as a response to simple trauma. However, the tendency to depapillation, even locally, is greatly increased in anaemias and related conditions in which the tongue epithelium is particularly liable to atrophic changes (**82**). More generalised depapillation is seen in anaemias, vitamin B12 and folate deficiencies (**83**), and is often accompanied by angular cheilitis (see Chapter 4). If the mouth is particularly dry—as, for instance, in Sjogren's syndrome, the filliform papillae may become in some areas atrophic and, in others, elongated and somewhat 'hairy' (**84**). This situation presumably reflects the non physiological oral environment (see Chapter 8). There is no evidence that atrophy of the papillae occurs as an age change uncomplicated by disease.

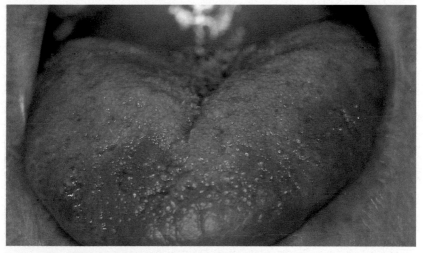

82 Depapillation of the tip and lateral margins of the tongue in a patient with undiagnosed pernicious anaemia.

Depapillation

Diagnosis: Initially clinical, laboratory investigations for haematological abnormalities.

Associated conditions: Anaemia, folate and vitamin B12 deficiency.

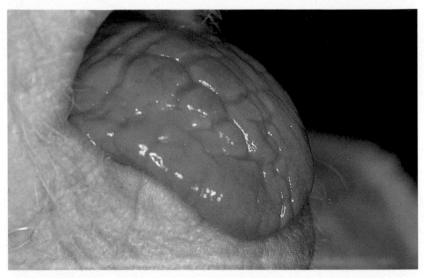

83 A widely depapillated tongue in a patient with a severe folate deficiency induced macrocytic anaemia showing the characteristic shiny surface.

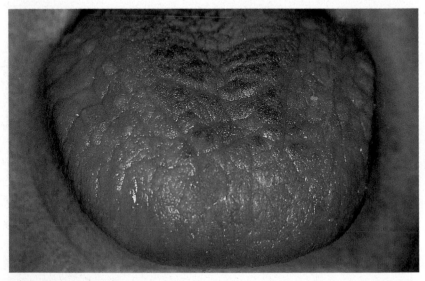

84 A dry tongue in a patient with Sjogren's syndrome. Some areas are slightly depapillated, others slightly 'hairy'.

Geographic tongue

Geographic tongue is a condition in which transient, patchy depapillation of the tongue occurs, leaving erythematous areas surrounded by a white border (**85**). The patches are said to resemble maps—hence the term 'geographic tongue'—whilst the Latin term *erythema migrans* indicates the apparent movement of the patches over the surface of the tongue. This simulated movement is due to the rapid appearance and disappearance of the lesions (over a few days) which start as small depapillated areas and then spread. The whole impression is that the lesions themselves are slowly moving over the surface. There is some variation in appearance and occasionally solitary lesions appear (**86**), which may be attributed to simple trauma (**87**). The lesions can also appear deceptively similar to other mucosal conditions—particularly, lichen planus (**88**). In general, however, the appearance and history of this condition are quite diagnostic. In general, the condition is asymptomatic, although there may be transient mild irritation—most patients are able to accept it as a 'normal' state. If, however, a previously pain-free condition becomes sore and irritable, consideration should be given to the possible onset of some condition (such as an anaemia or related condition) which might cause tongue soreness regardless of the presence of geographic patches. However, geographic tongue itself is not known to be associated with any other specific disease process. Its aetiology is quite unknown.

Geographic tongue

Diagnosis: Clinical.

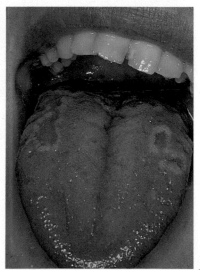

85 A typical geographic tongue.

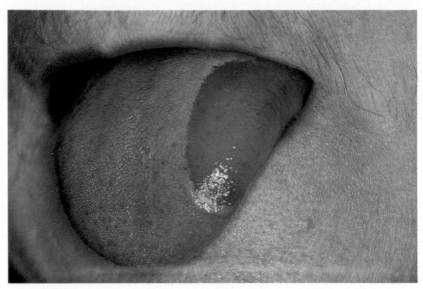

86 A solitary geographic patch on the lateral margin of the tongue.

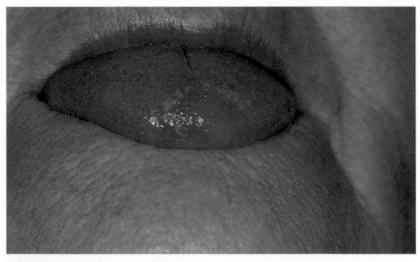

87 A geographic lesion of the tip of the tongue, easily mistakable for a mild traumatic lesion.

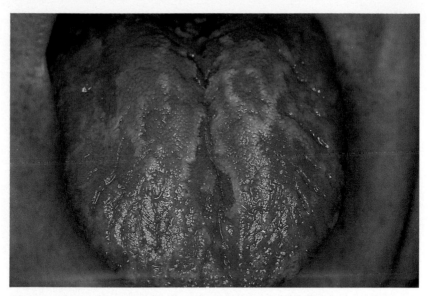

88 A tongue with geographic lesions simulating lichen planus.

Midline glossitis

Midline glossitis (median glossitis, median rhomboid glossitis) is a lesion of the midline of the tongue, which has a widely variable clinical presentation (**89, 90, 91**). Its aetiology is not clear, and for a long time it was thought to be a developmental condition. This is now considered not to be the case—it has never been reported in child patients. Current opinion holds that the lesion represents a response to chronic candidal infection. The lesion is responsive to prolonged antifungal treatment in some patients, but not in others. In some cases, there is a rather proliferative reaction around the midline (**92**), while in others, a proliferative midline lesion may cause concern as to the possibility of a neoplasm (**93**). The lesion, as initially described, forms a lozenge-shaped area at the site of the former embryonic tuberculum impar; it is, in fact, very uncommon (**94**). The lesions are quite symptom-free.

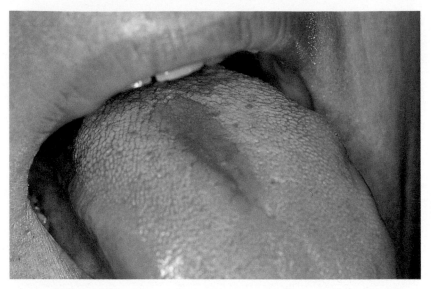

89, 90 and 91 (This page and top figure on facing page.) These illustrations show three of the more common of the wide range of presentations of midline glossitis.

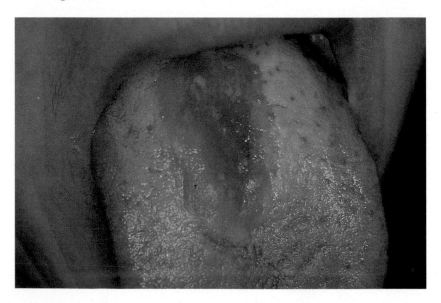

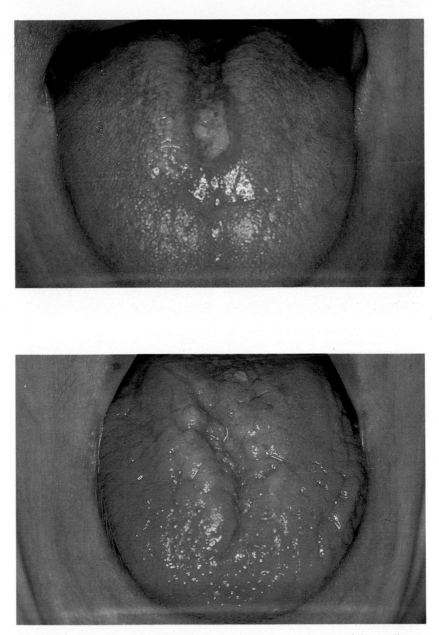

92 Midline glossitis with a proliferative reaction on each side of the midline.

71

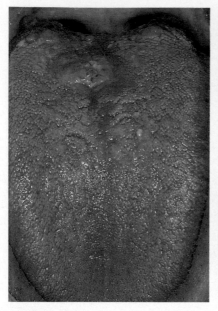 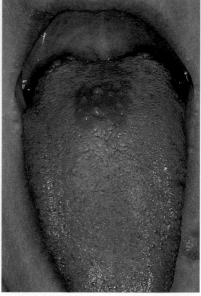

93 A proliferative midline form of midline glossitis.

94 The classic form of 'median rhomboid glossitis' as initially described.

Midline glossitis

Diagnosis: Clinical. Biopsy is not necessary, except in unusual circumstances.

Sore tongue

There are a considerable number of patients, predominantly older and female, who complain of a sore, irritated or burning tongue in the complete absence of any visible abnormality. This often represents a stage in the development of the so-called burning mouth syndrome (BMS), in which a sensation of soreness or burning affects the

whole mouth without any evident cause. In the making of this diagnosis, the possibility of early and subclinical changes attributable to
generalised disease must be kept in mind. A denture-related problem,
or some other source of chronic oral trauma, may be involved in
about half of the cases. Hormonal imbalance has often been quoted
as a possible aetiological factor for BMS, but there is no evidence to
support this. The evidence for allergy as a common cause of BMS is
equally weak. **Table 8** gives some of the possible causes of tongue
irritation to be considered in the differential diagnosis of sore tongue.

**TABLE 8   Some Possible Causes of Sore Tongue in the
Absence of Visible Signs**

Early generalised disease *
    Latent anaemias
    Folate, B12 deficiency
    Diabetes mellitus
    Rheumatoid arthritis
    Other connective tissue disease
    Sjogren's syndrome

Local irritation *
    Dentures, bridges, crowns
    Fractured tooth
    Mouthwashes
    Smoking
    Dry mouth (see above)
    Candidiasis

Burning mouth syndrome
    (no known physical cause)

Allergy rare

Hormonal imbalance rare

---

*   *Visible signs may appear later in these conditions.*

The Lips

As pointed out above, the lips may be the site of lesions in a wide range of conditions affecting the oral mucosa (see examples shown in Chapters 1, 2, 7, and 11). The vermillion border is usually involved in these cases, but in others (Chapters 1 and 7) the perioral skin seems particularly susceptible to the disease process. In just a few of the conditions the vermillion area of the lips only is affected, in the absence of either oral mucosal or skin lesions. In all lesions of this kind, an allergy to lipstick should be considered in the differential diagnosis.

Median lip fissures

Lip fissures—usually median, but occasionally away from the midline—are lesions which in most cases have no clear aetiology (**95**). In some instances they may be consequent on lip swelling, from whatever cause (**96**). The majority of these fissures are infected by *Staphylococcus aureus*, but some by *Candida* spp.

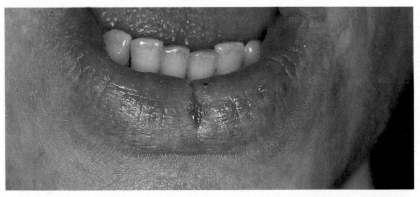

95 A persistent midline fissure of the lower lip, in this case infected by staphylococci.

Median lip fissures

Diagnosis: Clinical, laboratory culture of swabs to determine infecting organism prior to treatment.

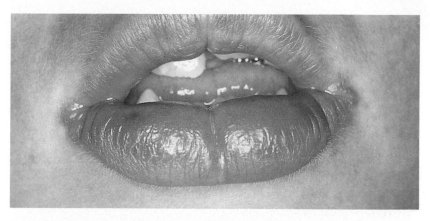

96 A midline fissure forming in the swollen lower lip of a patient with oral Crohn's disease.

Exfoliative cheilitis

This is a condition of unknown aetiology in which there is a grossly excessive production of keratin associated with increased mitotic activity in the basal layer of the epithelium. It is restricted to the vermillion border of the lips—predominantly the lower—and seems to be quite benign in its behaviour (**97**). It is periodic in nature, the affected lip becoming apparently normal in the intervening periods. The rest of the oral mucosa is completely unaffected. Most patients generally complain of no more than mild irritation, but in some patients, secondary infection and probable superimposed trauma from the teeth result in more crusted lesions (**98**). Although stress factors, atopy and self-inflicted trauma have been implicated, a fully credible explanation for the origin of this condition has not yet been given.

Exfoliative cheilitis

Diagnosis: Clinical, strongly dependant on history. Swabs to eliminate significant infection; biopsy not helpful.

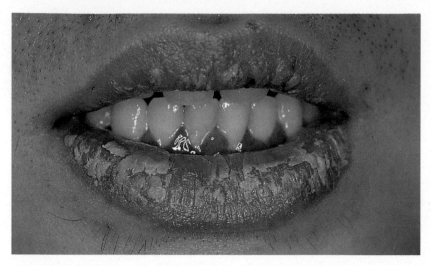

97 Exfoliative cheilitis showing the excessive formation of keratin.

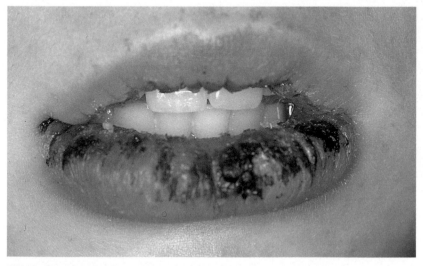

98 Exfoliative cheilitis, with some secondary trauma and infection.

Candidal cheilitis

Candidal cheilitis (candidal cheilosis, candido-cheilosis, cheilo - candidosis) is possibly related to exfoliative cheilitis, although this has not been proved. It is an uncommon condition in which ulcerated granulomatous lesions of the lips occur, heavily infected by *Candida* spp. (**99**). It has been suggested that sunlight may play a part as an initiating factor—a number of cases have been reported from Australia. However, not all recorded cases have occurred in predominantly sunny climates. It has also been suggested that, in the absence of vigorous treatment of the candidal infection, this condition should be considered as potentially malignant. There is, however, no real evidence for this.

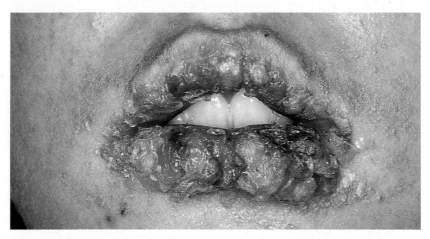

99 Candidal cheilitis showing heavily candida infected granulomatous lesions.

Candidal cheilitis

Diagnosis: Laboratory culture of swabs.

Important differential diagnosis: From (non-candidal) exfoliative cheilitis.

Actinic cheilitis

Actinic cheilitis (solar keratosis) occurs largely in male patients who have worked for long periods of time in strong sunlight. It predominantly affects the lower lip (**100**). The vermillion margin becomes crusted and indurated—this latter being due to a subepithelial fibrosis ('solar elastosis'). The epithelium may develop marked atypia which may progress, if untreated, to carcinoma—hence the term 'lip at risk'. Occasionally a similar condition may develop in patients who have not been exposed to excessive sunlight or who have been treated by ultra-violet light therapy. The steady progress of this condition marks it out as being quite different in behaviour from the two forms of cheilitis mentioned above.

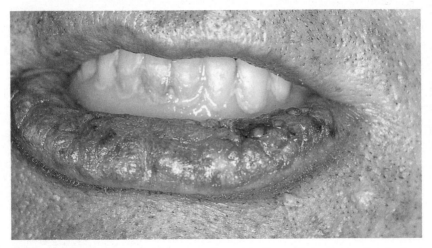

100 Actinic cheilitis—in this case, the epithelium of the lower lip showed marked atypia.

Actinic cheilitis

Diagnosis: Biopsy.

Lip swelling

The differential diagnosis of swellings affecting the lips is dealt with in Chapter 6.

Chapter 4

Disorders Of Blood And Nutrition

Oral signs and symptoms may appear in a wide range of disorders of the blood. These range from those which affect the erythrocytes and the iron transport mechanism, such as anaemias and vitamin or nutritional defiencies, and those affecting the leukocytes and platelcts, such as leukaemia, neutropenia and thrombocytopenia.

Anaemias and related conditions

Patients with anaemias, latent anaemias and associated conditions may present with a wide range of oral manifestations—the result of metabolic changes in the oral mucosa (see **Table 9**, overleaf). These oral changes are largely non-specific, and may occur in the early stages of the haematological disorder, often before the onset of alterations in the morphology of the erythrocytes. The oral changes in anaemias are closely linked with abnormalities in the nutritional factors which affect erythrocyte production—in particular, vitamin B12 and folic acid. Evidently, such abnormalities may be linked to disorders of nutrition or of the gastrointestinal tract. It is important to stress the following three factors:

- The oral changes are not specific to any particular haematological abnormality.

- The oral changes may occur in the early stages of the haematological abnormality and before they are detectable in a simple blood screen (haemoglobin, full blood count and film).

- As a result, an investigation should include estimates of serum B12, serum folate, red cell folate and serum ferritin levels, even in the presence of a normal haemoglobin level, full blood count and film.

However, it should be pointed out that some patients, even in advanced stages of haematological deficiency, show no oral changes of any kind.

TABLE 9 Oral Changes in Anaemias and Related Conditions*

Generalised stomatitis

	Burning mouth
	Gingivitis

Glossitis
Sore tongue
Depapillated tongue
Tongue unusually susceptible to trauma
Disturbances of taste

Ulceration
Recurrent oral ulceration
Non-specific ulceration

Candidiasis
Acute pseudomembranous candidiasis
Acute atrophic candidiasis
Angular cheilitis

Anaemias, latent anaemia, conditions associated with vitamin B12 or folate deficiency.

Anaemia

Uncomplicated iron deficiency is, perhaps, least likely to be the condition underlying major oral changes. In iron-depleted patients, the most common oral changes are angular cheilitis (**101, 102**) and depapillation of the tongue (**103**). A connection with recurrent oral ulceration is also less likely than in conditions involving folate or vitamin B12 deficiency. In the Plummer–Vinsun syndrome (also known as the Patterson–Kelly syndrome) there is an association between iron deficiency and dysphagia, often associated with the presence of an oesophageal web. There may be atrophy of the tongue papillae or, as in this case, areas of leukoplakia present on the tongue (**104**). Although well known, this is a relatively uncommon condition.

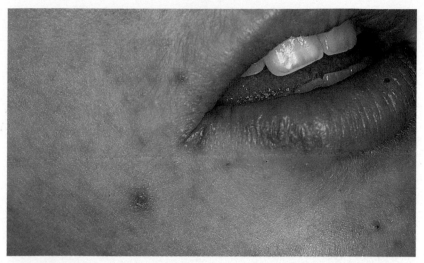

101 Angular cheilitis in a sixteen-year-old female patient with severe anaemia (haemoglobin 5g/dl). The anaemia was the result of excessive menstrual loss.

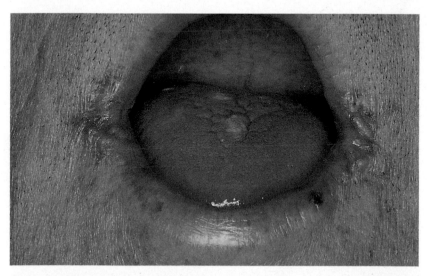

102 Angular cheilitis in a severely anaemic male patient. There are also patches of thrush visible on the dorsum of the tongue. The iron depletion was the result of gastrointestinal tract bleeding.

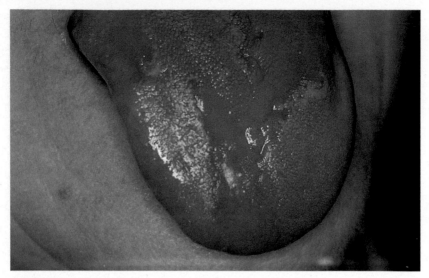

103 Patchy depapillation of the tongue in a patient with a much-reduced serum iron concentration—latent anaemia. The haemoglobin was within normal limits.

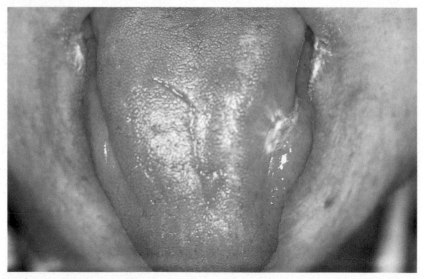

104 A leukoplakia on the tongue of a patient with Plummer–Vinsun syndrome.

Folate and B12 deficiencies

As pointed out in the preceding pages, deficiencies of folate or vitamin B12, however caused, may be responsible for any of the changes shown in **Table 9**. These two basic deficiencies cannot be differentiated on the basis of the oral signs and symptoms, as equivalent changes may occur in either.

The most common oral manifestations are of tongue depapillation (**105**) and angular cheilitis (**107**, **108**), although the other conditions mentioned in the table are regularly seen in these patients (**106**, **109** and **110**). In general, the oral effects of vitamin B12 and folate deficiency are more marked than in uncomplicated iron deficiency, particularly in the case of the discomfort arising from glossitis. The recurrence of aphthous ulceration in patients with folate and vitamin B12 deficiencies has been illustrated in Chapter 2 (Figure **63**). Some of the generalised conditions leading to folate and vitamin B12 deficiency are shown in **Table 10**.

TABLE 10 Some Causes of Folate and Vitamin B12 Deficiency	
Folate deficiency	Dietary
	Alcoholism
	Malabsorption states
	Pregnancy
	Drugs
	Anticonvulsants
	Cytotoxic
Vitamin B12 deficiency	Rarely dietary
	Pernicious anaemia
	Other malabsorption states
	Surgery to G.I.tract

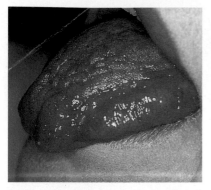

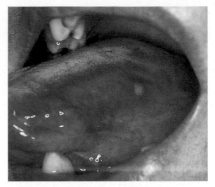

105 The shiny, red, depapillated tongue of a patient with severe folate deficiency.

106 Painful oral ulceration associated with folate deficiency due to malabsorption. These ulcers did not follow the pattern of recurrent oral ulceration (compare with Figure **63**).

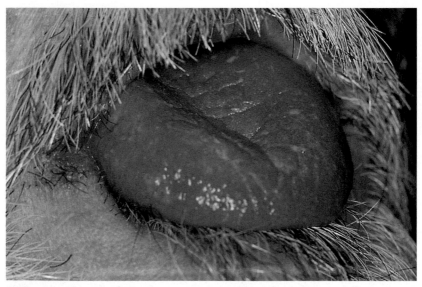

107 Angular cheilitis in a patient with marked folate deficiency of dietary/alcoholic origin. There are also flecks of pseudomembranous candidiasis visible on the tongue.

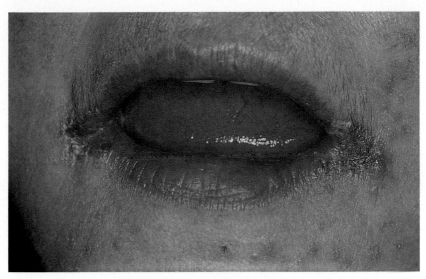

108 Marked angular cheilitis associated with pernicious anaemia. The tip of a sore and depapillated tongue is also visible.

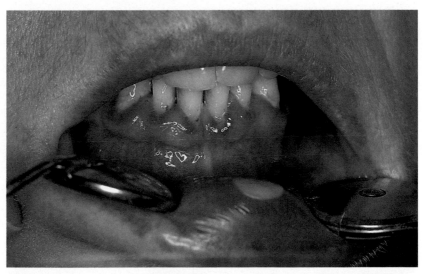

109 A patient with a complex malabsorption syndrome leading to much lowered serum folate and B12 levels and a consequent macrocytic anaemia. There is a generalised stomatitis, gingivitis and ulceration.

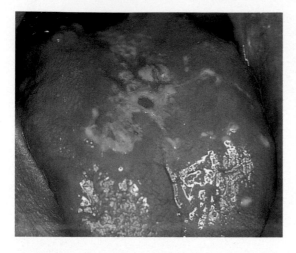

110 A patient who had undergone gastrectomy without follow-up replacement therapy. He was markedly deficient in iron, vitamin B12 and folate. Chronic pseudo-membranous candidiasis is present on the tongue. Patches of chronic hyperplastic candidiasis were present below the superficial plaques.

Other nutritional deficiencies

There are few specific oral changes described as commonly occurring in other vitamin deficiencies apart from those mentioned above. The changes described in other vitamin B group deficiencies are similar to those in folate and B12 deficiency. An exception to this is the effect of vitamin C deficiency on the oral cavity. In this condition (scurvy), the characteristic oral change is gingivitis, the papillae being swollen and fragile (**111**). The role of generalised malnutrition as a cause of secondary immunodeficiency and consequent problems has been illustrated in Chapter 1 (Figure **48**).

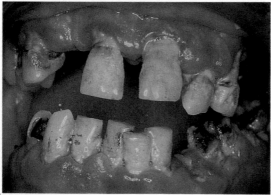

111 The characteristic picture in scurvy—a hyperplastic gingivitis complicated by neglected oral hygiene.

Leukaemias and related conditions

Leukaemia

Oral manifestations may be the first indication of acute leukaemia, and oral lesions can cause significant problems in the later stages of the disease. Although attempts have been made to differentiate between oral changes in the different forms of leukaemia, no generally accepted diagnostic indicators have been described.

The first oral indication of acute leukaemia may be a hyperplastic gingivitis, which in the early stages can be deceptively mild (**112**). Spontaneous gingival haemorrhage (**113**) or persistent acute ulcerative gingivitis are also early indicators of leukaemia. In the later stages of the disease, there may be widespread oral ulceration (**114**). These ulcers, formed by the breakdown of the mucosa overlying leukaemic deposits, can be very resistant to treatment (**115, 116**). A severe haemorrhagic and hypertrophic gingivitis is common (**117, 118**).

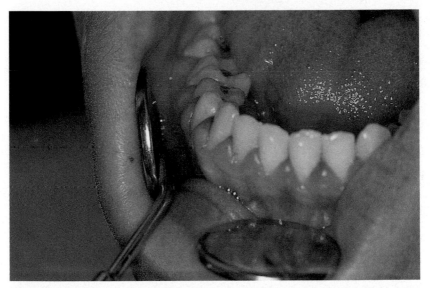

112 A mild hyperplastic gingivitis with minimal bleeding—the first indication of acute myeloid leukaemia in this 22- year-old patient.

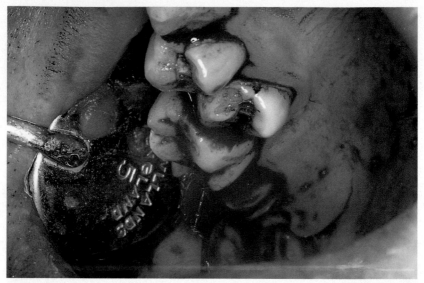

113 Spontaneous haemorrhage from the gingivae in acute lymphoblastic anaemia.

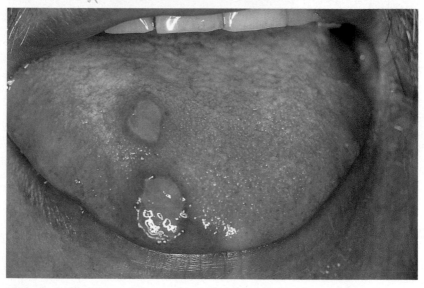

114 Oral ulceration in advanced lymphoblastic leukaemia.

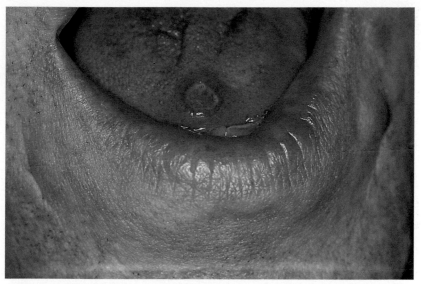

115 Oral ulcer in acute myeloid leukaemia caused by the breakdown of a leukaemic deposit similar to the skin lesion shown in **116**.

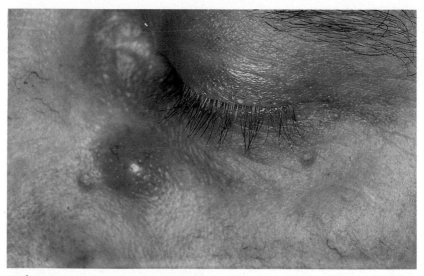

116 A skin deposit of leukaemic cells in the patient shown in **115**.

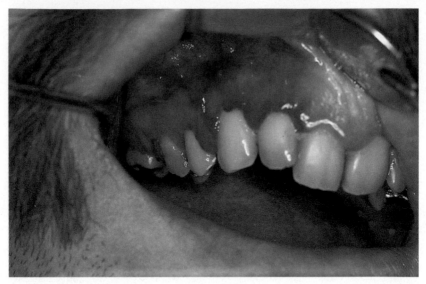

117 A marked haemorrhagic gingivitis in advanced acute myeloid leukaemia.

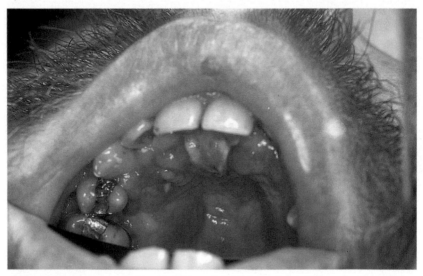

118 Hyperplastic palatal gingivitis, ulcerated in the midline, in the patient also shown in **117**.

Neutropenia

In severe neutropenia (agranulocytosis), the lack of protective granulocytes may lead to widespread infective episodes. It is often accompanied by severe oral ulceration (**119**). In cyclic neutropenia, a condition in which the number of circulating granulocytes varies widely, severe and painful oral ulceration may accompany the periods of neutropenia. These ulcers often heal with scarring (**120**).

119 Ulceration of the tongue in a patient with severe neutropenia.

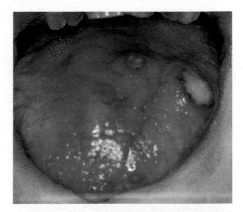

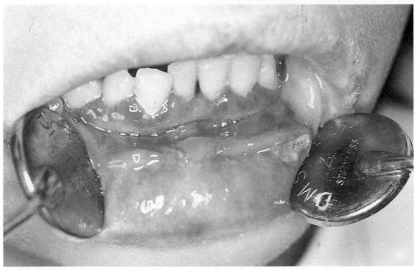

120 Scarring of the lower labial sulcus following ulceration in a young patient with cyclic neutropenia.

Thrombocytopenia

Thrombocytopenia—a reduction in the number of circulating platelets—may be revealed at an early stage by the appearance of petechial haemorrhages in the oral mucosa (**121**). In some patients, blood-filled bullae form on the mucosa, particularly as a response to trauma (**122**). A few patients may experience a similar reaction to mild trauma (i.e. the production of blood-filled bullae) in the absence of any platelet abnormality. These 'idiopathic blood blisters' have also been described by the unsatisfactory title 'angina bullosa haemorrhagica'—the word 'angina' referring to the pain sometimes experienced by the patients as the bullae form. Oral mucosal petechae may also be seen in generalised conditions in which the clotting mechanism of the blood is disturbed (**123**). Occasionally, the skin is also involved (**124**).

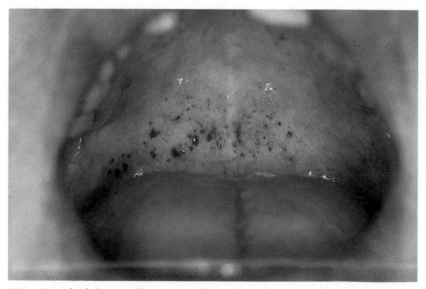

121 Petechial haemorrhages on the palate of a patient with idiopathic thrombocytopenia.

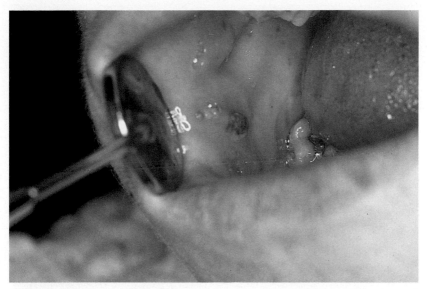

122 In this patient with thrombocytopenia, mild trauma of the buccal mucosa on the occlusal line has caused a small blood-filled bulla to form.

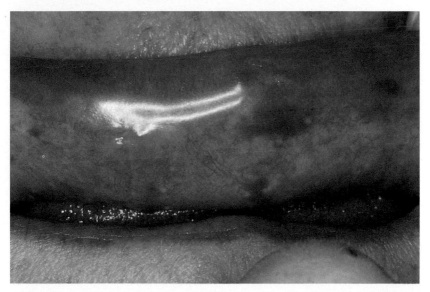

123 Mucosal petechae in a patient with clotting defects secondary to amyloidosis.

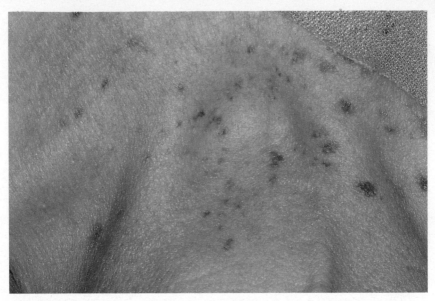

124 Skin lesions in the patient shown in **123**.

Thrombocytopenia

- **Diagnosis:** Haematology screen, including platelets and coagulation studies.

- **Important differential diagnosis:** From mucosal telangiectasia.

Chapter 5

Gastro-Intestinal Tract Disease

The mouth, as a part of the gastro-intestinal tract, may be involved in diseases affecting other parts of the tract. This involvement may be either primary—in which lesions similar to those in the lower gut appear in the mouth—or secondary. The most common secondary involvement is the result of malabsorption, with consequent changes in the oral mucosa such as those described in Chapter 4. Oral ulceration may occur in many patients with lower GI tract problems. This is often described as aphthous ulceration, although it often does not have the characteristics of recurrent aphthous ulceration as properly defined. Three conditions are of particular significance: coeliac disease and the two inflammatory bowel diseases, ulcerative colitis and Crohn's disease.

Table 11 (overleaf) summarises the oral features in these three gastro-intestinal tract diseases. See Chapter 11 for Peutz–Jegher's syndrome (multiple intestinal polyps associated with circumoral melanotic pigmentation).

Crohn's.

Coeliac disease

Coeliac disease (gluten enteropathy) represents an immunological response to the protein gluten in the diet. Many patients with established coeliac disease are known to suffer from oral ulceration or a generalised stomatitis as part of the disease pattern. This includes the failure to thrive in children, and major digestive disturbances in all ages. It has only recently become evident that recurrent oral ulceration may be the only symptom shown by some patients who display the typical changes of coeliac disease in the jejeunum.

These changes, precipitated by the dietary gluten, consist of partial or total atrophy of the jejeunal villi, with some underlying inflammatory changes and hyperplasia of the crypts (**125, 126**). If gluten is withdrawn from the diet, these changes reverse and the oral ulceration disappears. Patients may have no symptoms suggestive of coeliac disease other than recurrent oral ulceration. This may be of any of the three recognised types described in Chapter 2, but is most commonly minor aphthous or herpetiform ulceration (**127**). All such reported patients have been adults; but it is not clear at what point the jejeunal abnormality develops in patients of this kind. Only a small pro-

TABLE 11   Oral Manifestations in Gastro-intestinal Tract Disease

Coeliac disease	ROU (specific link)
	Ulceration (non-ROU)
	Candidiasis
	Changes due to malabsorption
Ulcerative colitis	Ulceration (ROU and non-ROU)
	Candidiasis
	Pyostomatitis gangrenosum
	Pyostomatitis vegetans
	Changes due to malabsorption
Crohn's disease	Ulceration (ROU and non-ROU)
	Swollen lips and cheeks
	Angular cheilitis
	Palpable lymph nodes
	Buccal irregularities
	Gingivitis

ROU = recurrent oral ulceration (Chapter 2)
*Changes due to malabsorption summarised in **Table 9***

portion of patients with recurrent oral ulceration fall into this cate-gory—4% at the most is the probable figure—although some sur-veys of selected groups have suggested a higher level. A definitive diagnosis can be made only after jejeunal biopsy has confirmed vil-lous atrophy. The selection of patients for biopsy depends on the demonstration of indications of malabsorption in a full haematology screen: a reduction in haemoglobin, serum iron, serum or red cell folate or vitamin B12 levels.

In patients with the classical form of coeliac disease, the distur-bance of calcium metabolism at weaning may result in a band-like line of hypoplasia in the teeth calcifying at that time (see Chapter 13). In a few patients, coeliac disease may be difficult to control, even by strict dietary regimes, and there may be a secondary immune defi-ciency leading to oral infections of the kind described in Chapter 1. Oral ulceration may be severe, and may be accompanied by the skin lesions of dermatitis herpetiformis—also a coeliac disease–related condition (**128**).

125 A section of normal jejunal mucosa with well developed villi.

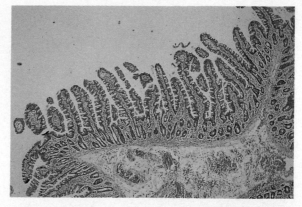

126 A section of jejunal mucosa from a patient with coeliac disease, showing villous atrophy. The magnification is the same as that of **125**.

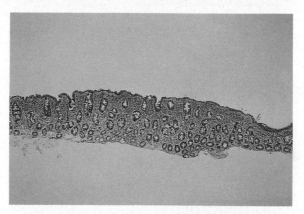

Coeliac disease

Diagnosis: Full haematology screening, jejunal biopsy.

Associated conditions: Dermatitis herpetiformis.

Important differential diagnosis: From ROU not associated with systemic disease.

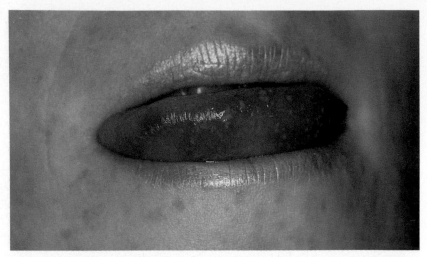

127 Herpetiform ulceration in a female patient, aged 24, who was found to have a flat jejunal mucosa on biopsy. The ulceration went into remission on a gluten-free diet.

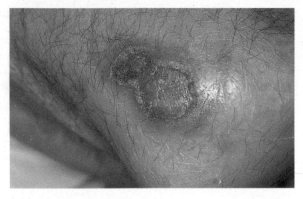

128 Skin lesions in a patient with coeliac disease and persistent oral ulceration.

Ulcerative colitis

In some patients with ulcerative colitis, the inflammatory and ulcerative changes taking place in the colon are accompanied by oral ulceration. These oral ulcers may be persistent and destructive, even when relatively small (**129**). In other patients—usually those with very active colonic disease—the oral ulcers may be large (pyostomatitis gangenosum, **130**) and resemble the aggressive skin lesions (pyoderma gangrenosum) which occur in similar circumstances. These lesions heal with scarring (**131**, **132**). A less-active lesion (pyostomatitis vegitans) is also the oral equivalent of a skin lesion (pyostomatitis vegitans), in which numbers of small microabscesses are contained in a granular lesion (**133**, **134**). These oral lesions are not specific to ulcerative colitis, as they have been described in patients with other forms of large bowel disease.

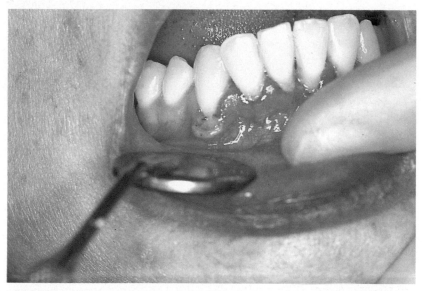

129 A small but persistent and painful ulcer on the gingival margin in a patient with active ulcerative colitis.

Ulcerative colitis

Diagnosis: Clinical (history highly significant). Oral biopsy is only occasionally necessary.

Associated conditions: Skin lesions (pyoderma) in severely affected patients.

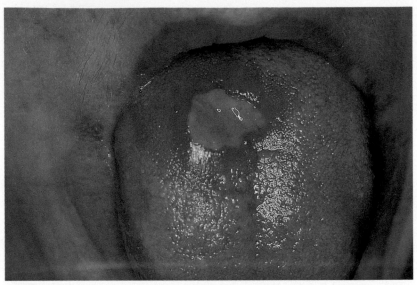

130 Pyostomatitis gangrenosum affecting the midline of the tongue.

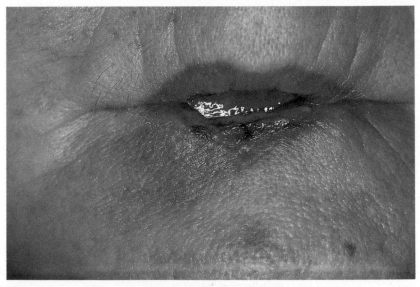

131 Pyostomatitis gangrenosum affecting the lower lip.

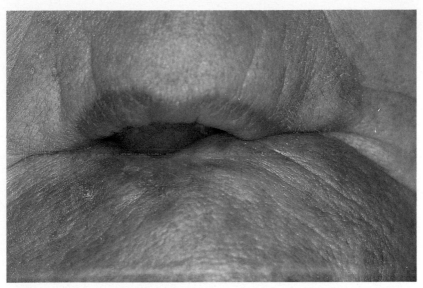

132 The lip of the patient in **131**, showing residual deformity after healing.

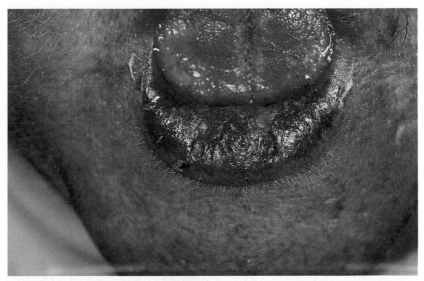

133 Pyostomatitis vegitans affecting the lower lip.

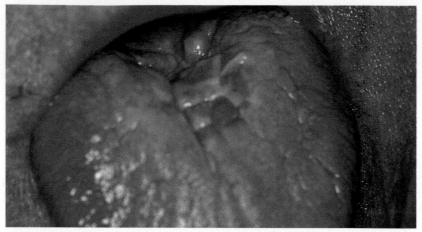

134 Pyostomatitis vegetans in the midline of the tongue.

Crohn's disease

Crohn's disease was first described in 1932, with the possibility of oral lesions being reported in the late 1960s. Since then, there have been many reports. Crohn's disease may occur at any site in the gastro-intestinal tract—including the oral cavity. The oral manifestations are exactly parallel with those in other sites: mucosal inflammation and ulceration (**135**); lymph node changes leading to obstructive oede-ma—most commonly of the lips (**136**) and occasionally of the cheeks (**137**)—and the production of granulomas lying within folds; and irregularities in the buccal and labial tissues (**138**) and the gingivae. These granulomas have a characteristic non-caseating tuberculoid structure (**139**). The angular cheilitis occurring in oral Crohn's disease is primary, and may occur in the absence of lip swelling. It is analo-gous to the anal fissures which occur in anal Crohn's disease. The changes in the cervical lymph nodes cause them to become firm and palpable, but not tender.

Oral lesions may occur before, with, or after the recognition of generalised Crohn's disease, and thus may be an important diagnostic feature. It is undoubtedly true that many patients are now known with oral changes only, without any diagnosed disease in other parts of the gastro-intestinal tract. Although it is inevitable that a number of these will eventually develop such more widespread disease, the term 'oro-facial granulomatosis' has been coined to describe the disease active only in the single site. This situation will be further described in Chapter 6.

135 An ulcer in the buccal sulcus of a patient with generalised Crohn's disease. The diagnosis was made after biopsy of the margins of the ulcer showed non-caseating tuberculoid granulomatous tissue.

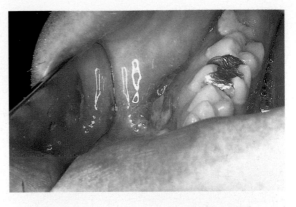

136 Lip swelling in a patient with established Crohn's disease.

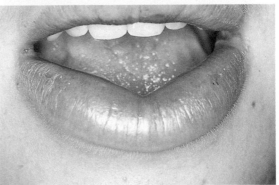

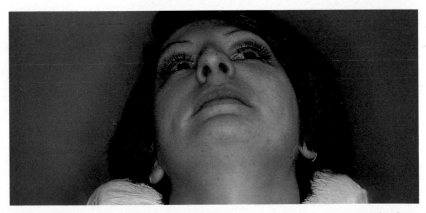

137 Swelling of the cheek in a patient with oral Crohn's disease, who later developed Crohn's lesions in the colon.

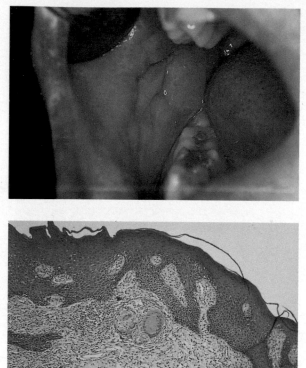

138 Folds in the buccal mucosa, containing characteristic granulomas in a patient with active gut Crohn's disease.

139 A section of a non-caseating tuberculoid granuloma in a buccal biopsy taken from a patient with oral Crohn's disease.

Crohn's disease

Diagnosis: Clinical picture suggestive only. Biopsy of oral granulomas*, haematological screen for malabsorption, contrast radiography, endoscopy/biopsy.

* Biopsy should be of buccal lesion if possible—biopsy of swollen lip is likely to show only oedema.

Important differential diagnosis: From other causes of swollen lip (see Chapter 6).

Granulomatous Diseases

In this chapter several diverse conditions, largely of unknown aetiology, are brought together, the common factor being that granuloma formation is prominent in each disease process. This arrangement does not imply any kind of common basis for these widely varied diseases. The conditions may be divided into two groups: those producing non-caseating tuberculoid granulomas, and those producing other types.

'Tuberculoid granulomatous disease'

A spectrum of oral conditions has been described in which tuberculoid granulomas may be involved. The precise definitions of these conditions are not established, and the 'spectrum' concept is generally accepted. There are, however, some fairly well-delineated clinical pictures which are described in the following.

Oro-facial granulomatosis

Oro-facial granulomatosis (OFG) is a term which has been introduced to define the condition described in Chapter 5 as oral Crohn's disease in the absence of more generalised Crohn's lesions. A term previously employed—cheilitis granulomatosa—probably also refers to this condition. A role for hypersensitivity in the aetiology of OFG has been postulated, but is not yet proven. All illustrations of OFG in this chapter could equally apply to oral Crohn's disease (i.e. oral lesions in the presence of generalised Crohn's lesions). An as yet unknown proportion of these patients will eventually develop Crohn's disease in other parts of the gastro-intestinal tract.

Lip swelling with angular cheilitis is the most common complaint (**140**); midline lip fissures may also occur (**141**), and the lip swelling may be gross (**142**). Angular cheilitis is a primary feature, and may occur in the absence of lip swelling (**143**). The skin overlying the swollen lip may, in some patients, be erythematous and scaly (**144**). Fissuring and irregularity of the buccal mucosa is usual, with the abnormal tissue containing the tuberculoid granulomas (**145**). A granular gingivitis is common (**146**); on biopsy, the affected gingival tissue is also found to contain granulomas. However, not all these features may be present in a single patient.

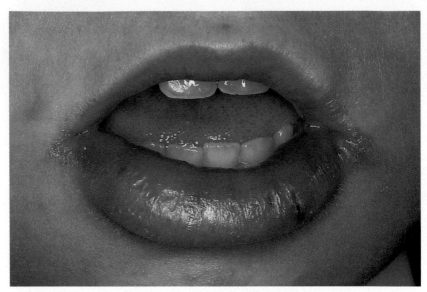

140 Swelling of the lower lip with angular cheilitis in OFG.

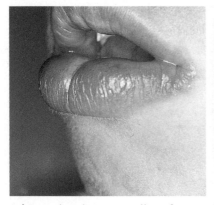

141 A developing midline fissure affecting a swollen lip in OFG.

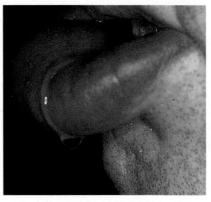

142 Gross swelling of the lower lip in OFG.

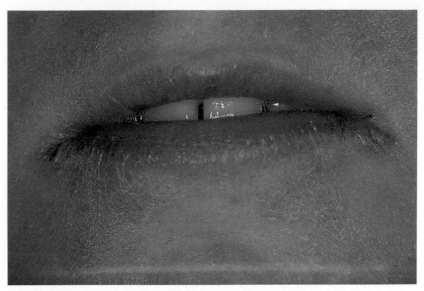

143 Angular cheilitis in OFG in the absence of lip swelling.

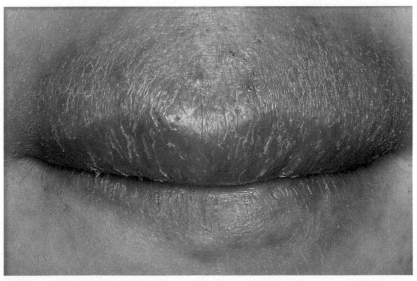

144 Erythema and scaling of the perioral skin in OFG.

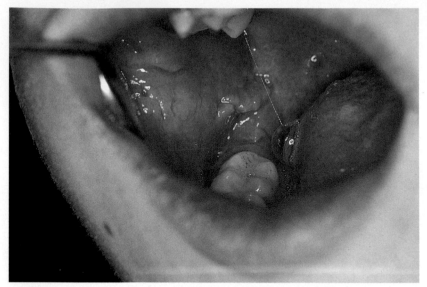

145 Irregular buccal mucosa in OFG. Biopsy showed characteristic granuloma formation.

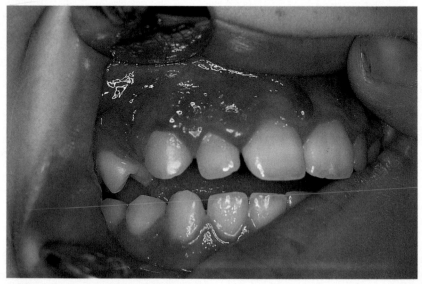

146 Granulomatous gingivitis in OFG.

Oro-facial granulomatosis

Diagnosis: Clinical, confirmed by biopsy of irregular mucosa, not of oedematous lip. Biopsy should be down to muscle, with some granulomas deeply sited. Investigations as for oral Crohn's disease: eliminate generalised involvement if suspected. Patch testing for hypersensitivity; value not yet determined.

Important differential diagnosis: From oral manifestations of generalised Crohn's disease and other causes of swollen lip.

Melkersson–Rosenthal syndrome

In this relatively rare but well-documented condition, the features of oro-facial granulomatosis, as described above, are present, together with an associated paralysis of the facial nerve (intermittent and in some cases bilateral) and a deeply midline fissured tongue (**147**). To these should be added intermittent facial pain of a migrainous type (this additional component has been described in several reports). The aetiology of this strangely diverse syndrome is quite unknown.

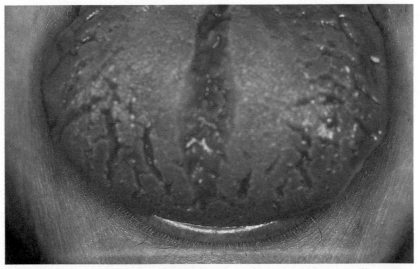

147 A deep midline tongue fissure in a patient with the Melkersson–Rosenthal syndrome.

Melkersson–Rosenthal syndrome

Diagnosis: Predominantly clinical. Biopsy as for OFG.

Sarcoidosis

Sarcoidosis is a granulomatous disease which may affect a number of organs, but predominantly the lungs and skin. The granulomas are of a non-caseating tuberculoid type, effectively indistinguishable from those in OFG. Diagnosis of sarcoid, in the presence of such granulomas, depends largely on the radiographic demonstration of lung involvement. Oral mucosal or perioral involvement is not common, but may occur (**148**, **149**). Lip swelling, as in Crohn's disease or OFG, is not a feature. The salivary glands may be involved; it has been shown that a considerable proportion of patients with the established disease are found on biopsy to have granulomas present in the labial mucous glands. The Kweim test (a granulomatous skin reaction to injected human sarcoid material) is said to be diagnostic, but may also be occasionally positive in Crohn's disease. This makes its use in the differential diagnosis of oral sarcoid from oral Crohn's disease somewhat problematic.

Sarcoidosis

Diagnosis: Dependent on biopsy, chest radiography, Kweim test (but see above).

Important differential diagnosis: From Crohn's disease, OFG.

Swollen lip

A list of some causes of swollen lip, to be considered in the differential diagnosis of oro-facial granulomatosis and Crohn's disease, is given in **Table 12** (page 112).

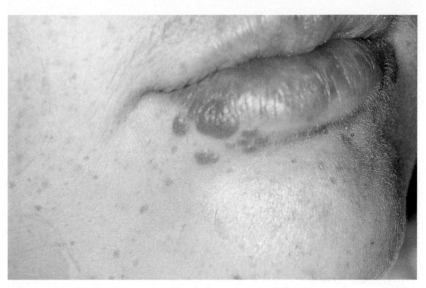

148 Lesions of the lips and perioral skin in sarcoidosis.

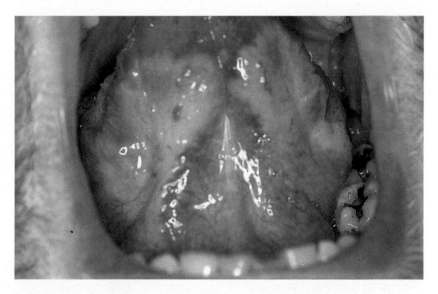

149 Lesions of sarcoidosis affecting the ventral surface of the tongue.

111

TABLE 12 Some Causes of Swollen Lip

Dental infection
> Acute abscess

Trauma
> Lip biting

Secondary to ulceration
> Major apthous ulceration
> Erythema multiforme

Allergy*
> Drugs
> Cosmetics
> Other allergens (e.g. plants)

Angio-oedema*

Crohn's disease

Oro-facial granulomatosis

Melkersson–Rosenthal syndrome

* Angio-oedema and allergies—see Chapter 12.

Non-tuberculoid granulomatous disease

Wegener's granulomatosis

Wegener's granulomatosis is representative of a spectrum of destructive granulomatous vasculitic diseases which may affect various organs—in particular, the upper respiratory tract, the lungs, the kidneys and the skin (**150**). There may also be ulcerated oral lesions (**151**). The most characteristic oral manifestation of Wegener's granulomatosis is a granulomatous gingivitis (**152**), which has a virtually diagnostic appearance. It does not appear in every case, however. The oral manifestations in related diseases (lethal midline granuloma, polyarteritis nodosa, etc.) are less clearly defined.

150 A destructive lesion of Wegener's granulomatosis on the skin of the thigh.

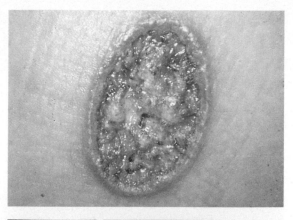

151 A buccal ulcerative lesion in Wegener's granulomatosis.

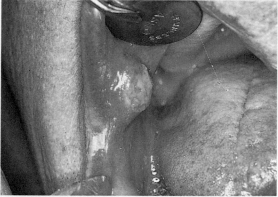

152 The characteristic gingivitis of Wegener's granulomatosis.

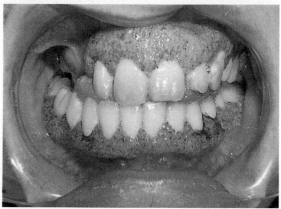

Histiocytoses

The histiocytoses (histiocytosis X, Langerhans' cell histiocytoses) are a group of conditions resulting from uncontrolled (but not malignant) proliferation of Langerhans' leukocytes to produce lesions in various sites. The resulting entities have been grouped according to the differing clinical pictures (eosinophilic granuloma, Letterer–Siwe disease and Hand–Schuller–Christian disease are some of the terms which have been used). The oral significance of these conditions is that the sites of infiltration of the abnormal cells may include the gingivae and alveolar bone, with consequent rapid local tissue destruction (**153**).

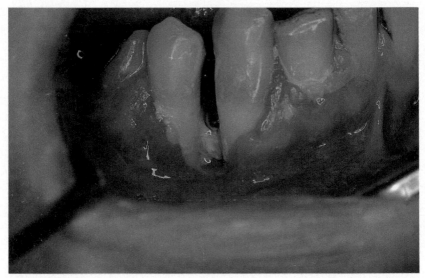

153 Gross gingival and alveolar bone destruction in histiocytosis.

Histiocytoses

Diagnosis: All histiocytoses—dependent on full clinical study with biopsy. Immunological findings not clearly defined.

Chapter 7

Diseases Of The Skin

The histological structure of the oral mucosa is that of a typical lining mucous membrane, but its behaviour often parallels that of the skin—thus a number of essentially dermatological diseases result in oral mucosal lesions.

It is not easy to explain why some skin diseases frequently result in oral lesions, whilst others do not. Oral lichen planus is a common condition, and a high proportion of patients with this generalised disease develop oral lesions. By contrast, psoriasis—an even more common skin disease than lichen planus—has never been convincingly shown to produce specific oral changes. In some skin diseases the oral lesions may be the first to appear, often by a substantial interval, and may be of particular importance in diagnosis. Pemphigus is an example of this, as the recognition of the oral lesions which precede skin lesions may lead to the early institution of treatment in this potentially fatal condition.

Although the initial diagnosis in this group of conditions is evidently based on clinical features, mucosal biopsy may be essential to arrive at a definitive diagnosis. Immunofluorescent technique may be particularly valuable in some, but not all, cases. While in some conditions (for instance, lichen planus) the oral lesions may bear little clinical resemblance to those of the skin, the histological features are shared by the skin and mucosal lesions. Other mucosae may also be involved in the skin diseases which affect the oral mucosa; for instance, genital lichen planus is by no means uncommon, and may occur at the same time as oral lichen planus. The coexistence of oral and genital mucosal symptoms should always be considered as an indicator of the possibility that the same process may be affecting both sites.

Lichen planus

Lichen planus is a disease of skin and mucous membranes which is relatively common, and is often seen in the oral medicine clinic. In patients reporting with skin lesions, some 70% are found to have oral lesions, whereas among those reporting primarily with oral lesions, only 35% are found to have skin lesions. This apparent inconsistency depends on the relatively asymptomatic nature of many of the oral lesions—they are not noticed by the patient, and are thus not investigated.

Another reason for discrepancies in the figures depends on the fact that the onset of skin and mucosal lesions may be widely separated in time. The duration of skin lesions alone is relatively short—the average is nine months. However, when mucosal lesions are involved, the duration may be much longer—several years is not uncommon. The age range at first presentation of patients with oral lesions is very wide, and may include children under the age of ten years. This would be considered very unusual in the case of skin lesions only. There is a female preponderance (70%) of patients presenting because of oral lesions, contrasting with 54% reported to attend for treatment of skin lesions. Also, there is a wide range of oral lesions in lichen planus, none of which resemble the typical skin lesions (**154**) but all of which share a very similar histological appearance (**155**). Lesions of the facial skin (**156**) are very rare, but scalp lesions are more common (**157**). It is convenient to classify the lesions of oral lichen planus into the following three groups: non-erosive, minor erosive and major erosive.

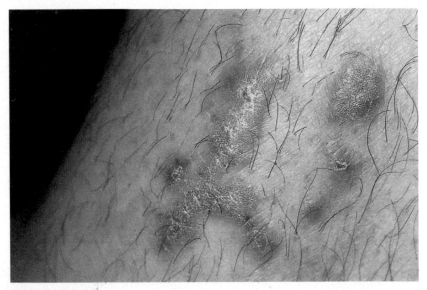

154 Typical skin lesions of lichen planus on the flexor surface of the wrist— pink-to-purple papules with white streaks on their surface (Wickham's striae).

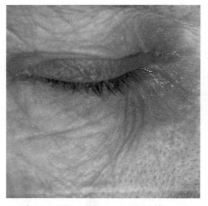

155 The characteristic histological appearance of lichen planus of all types—mucosal or skin. The dominant feature is a wide cellular band (largely of lymphocytes) lying in the corium. Whatever the clinical variant, this histology is usually recognisable.

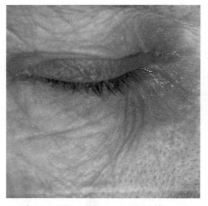

156 Lichen planus affecting the inner canthus of the eye.

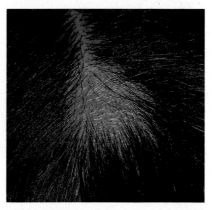

157 A patch of alopecia associated with a scalp lesion of lichen planus.

Non-erosive lichen planus

Non-erosive lichen planus characteristically appears as a reticular pattern of white streaks on the oral mucosa (**158**, **159** and **160**). The lesions are quite pain-free, and are often noticed coincidentally. Any part of the mucosa may be affected, but rarely the soft palate. In some patients the lesions may be confluent, and may resemble a leukoplakia (**161** and **162**; see Chapter 9 for comparative lesions). In these cases, however, there are almost always some areas which retain some degree of reticular pattern (**163**). In some instances the lesions may be concentrated in areas of the mucosa, suggesting a traumatic co-factor in their production (**164**).

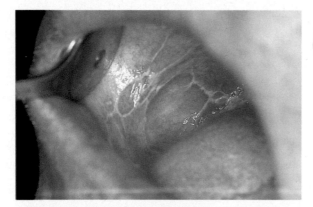

158 A typical reticular pattern in non-erosive lichen planus.

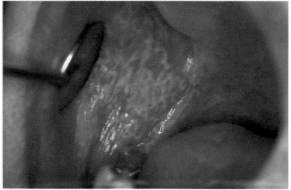

159 A variant of the reticular pattern in non-erosive lichen planus, as equally characteristic as that in **158**.

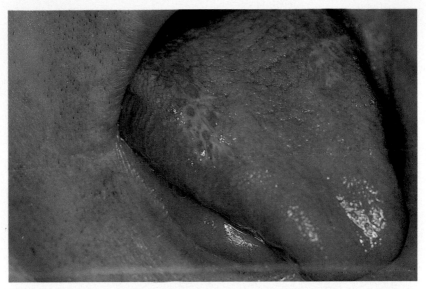

160 A slightly modified reticular pattern as frequently seen on the tongue in lichen planus.

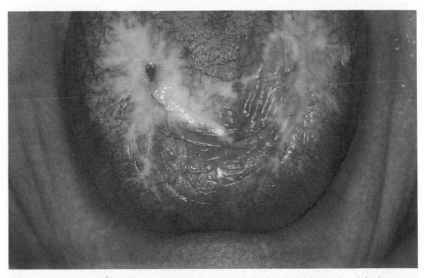

161 A dense white lesion on the tongue with the histology (and behaviour pattern) of lichen planus.

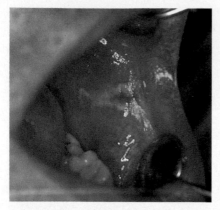

162 A lesion of lichen planus of the buccal mucosa with a strong resemblance to a commissural leukoplakia.

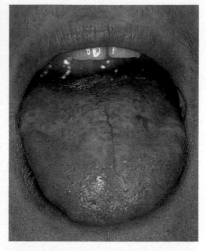

163 A lesion of lichen planus on the tongue, largely confluent, but with some reticular features at its margins.

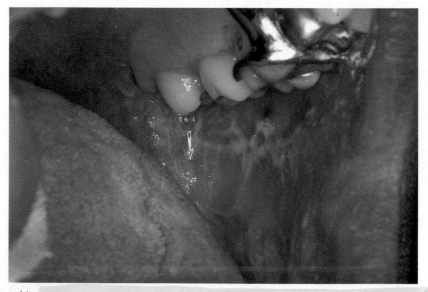

164 Lesions of lichen planus lying along the occlusal plane of the buccal mucosa.

Minor erosive lichen planus

In minor erosive lichen planus, some areas of the epithelium become atrophic and are lost with the formation of erosions (**165** and **166**). These lesions, unlike the non-erosive form, may give considerable discomfort. Frequently, the gingivae are also involved (**167**). The resulting desquamative gingivitis may, in fact, be the only oral manifestation of lichen planus—a parallel situation obtains in the case of pemphigoid, and clinical differentiation between these two may be difficult. In some patients the gingivae may appear as erythematous, without the erosive areas or white striae which might, in other sites, suggest a clinical diagnosis of lichen planus (**168** and **169**).

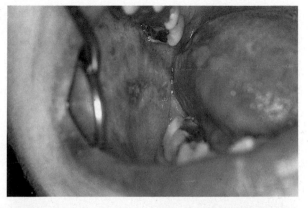

165 Minor erosive lichen planus of the buccal mucosa.

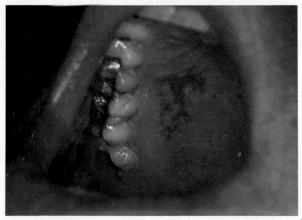

166 Minor erosive lichen planus of the palatal mucosa. The site is unusual, but not rare.

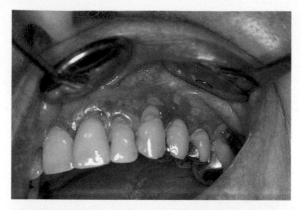

167 Erosive lichen planus of the gingivae.

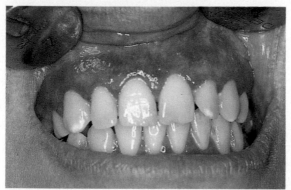

168 Erythematous diffuse lesions of lichen planus affecting the gingivae without erosions or white striae.

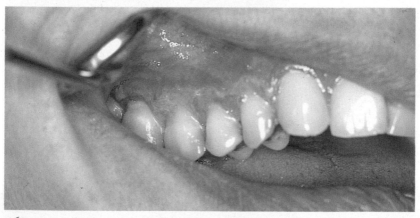

169 Gingival non-erosive lichen planus with evident white striae.

Major erosive lichen planus

In major erosive lichen planus, the characteristic lesions are remarkably different from those of the minor erosive form. The erosions present as clearly defined ulcers, covered by a raised yellow plaque with a glazed appearance (**170**). In some instances, large areas of mucosa may be involved in the erosive process (**171**). Although the clinical appearance is highly specific, confirmation by biopsy from an eroded lesion may be difficult. However, even when the erosions are widespread, there is almost always a non-erosive area present and available for biopsy—often on the lip mucosa (**172**). The lip may also be affected by erosive lesions which are susceptible to trauma and may appear in a form quite different from that of other major erosions (**173**). With the degeneration of the basal layer of the epithelium in lichen planus there is a mechanical weakening of the dermal–epidermal junction. Usually this leads to loss of the epithelium to form an erosion, but rarely the epithelium may lift intact to form bullae (**174**). These bullae are short-lived, disintegrating to form erosions, and as a result, bullous lichen planus rarely continues as such for any appreciable length of time (**175**).

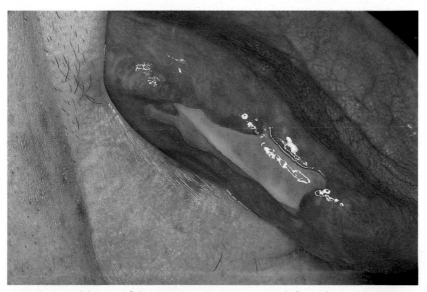

170 A typical lesion of the tongue in major erosive lichen planus.

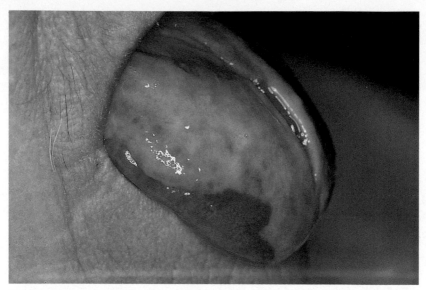

171 A lesion of major erosive lichen planus affecting most of the dorsal surface of the tongue.

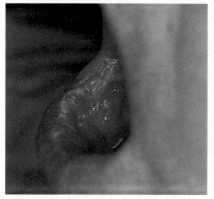

172 A non-erosive lesion of lichen planus on the lower lip of a patient with otherwise major erosive lesions—the patient shown in **171**.

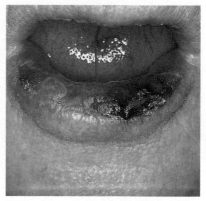

173 Crusting of the lower lip caused by trauma from the teeth on a major erosive lesion of lichen planus.

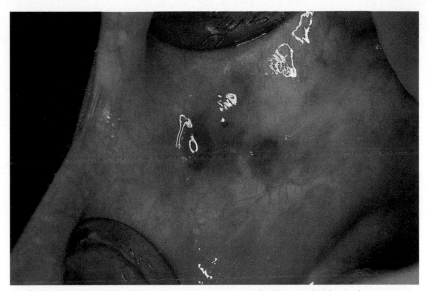

174 Bullous lichen planus showing an intact bulla on the buccal mucosa—an unusual situation.

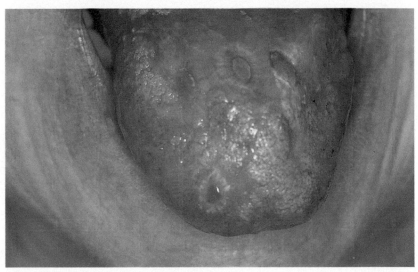

175 Bullous lichen planus in which the short-lived bullae have mostly disintegrated, leaving circular erosions on the tongue.

Melanotic reactive deposits and lichen planus

Following the resolution of the keratotic lesions of lichen planus, a melanotic reactive deposit in the underlying dermis may become visible (**176**). Such deposits may also form in relation to other white mucosal lesions, including leukoplakias, but do not have any diagnostic or prognostic significance.

There has been much discussion as to the pre-malignant potential of oral lichen planus. If strict criteria are applied to the initial diagnosis of lichen planus, the acceptable case reports are relatively few. Nonetheless, the possibility of malignant transformation in a previously established area of lichen planus does exist (**177** and **178**). A figure of a maximum of 1% or so of all cases is suggested as a reasonable estimate, although some (less well-documented) surveys have suggested a higher figure.

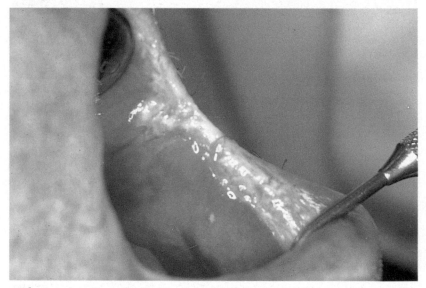

176 A melanotic residual area of the buccal mucosa following partial resolution of a lesion of non erosive lichen planus.

177 A squamous cell carcinoma of the buccal mu-cosa, arising in an area of lichen planus eight years after histologically confirmed diagnosis as such.

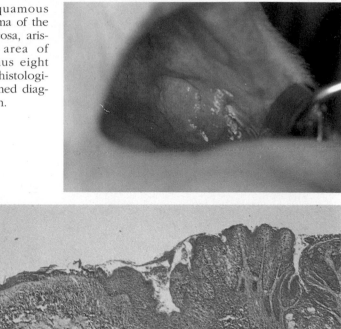

178 A section of the biopsy taken from the lesion shown in **177**. There are still some characteristic features of lichen planus visible in the non carcinomatous area of the section.

Lichen Planus

Diagnosis: Biopsy. Immunofluorescence does not give positive results for LP.

Important differential diagnosis: From connective tissue diseases (see chapter 8).

Lichenoid reactions

Lichen planus, including any of its oral forms, may be precipitated as a reaction to a wide range of drugs—the so-called 'lichenoid reaction'. It may be difficult to determine in some cases whether there is, in fact, drug involvement, as the condition does not necessarily subside immediately upon withdrawal of the drug. Some of the drugs most commonly involved in lichenoid reactions are listed in **Table 13**, although many others have been reported as being occasionally responsible.

TABLE 13 Lichenoid Reactions and Erythema Multiforme: Some Precipitating Factors

Lichenoid reactions	*Drugs**
	NSAIDs
	Gold salts
	Penicillamine
	Carbamazepine
	Methyldopa
	Some β-blockers
Erythema multiforme	*Infections*
	Herpes simplex
	Influenza
	Other viral infections
	Drugs*
	Barbiturates
	Sulphonamides
	Carbamazepine
	Penicillins
	Some NSAIDs, including:
	Fenbufen
	Phenylbutazone

---

* Many other drugs have been recorded as having occasionally caused lichenoid reactions or erythema multiforme.

Bullous diseases

In this group of disorders, lesions present initially in the form of bullae (blisters) caused by the collection of fluid below the epithelium or between its cells. Many patients have oral as well as skin lesions—in pemphigus, in particular, the oral lesions may precede others by a considerable interval. Diagnosis on the basis of oral lesions is quite possible, and may lead to suppression of the incipient skin bullae by early treatment. In this group of diseases the oral bullae tend to rupture with mild trauma, leaving erosions as the most prominent feature (**179–182**). It may, in fact, be difficult in some cases to identify the

179 Sub-eithelial bullous lesion.

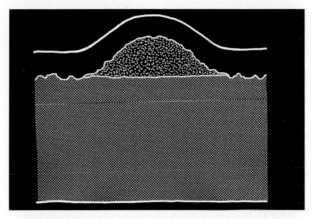

180 Intra-epithelial bullous lesion.

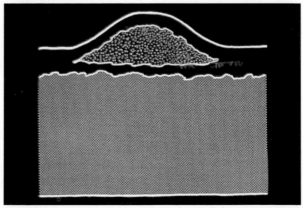

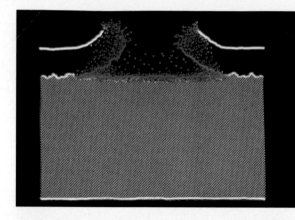

181 and 182 (below) Bullous lesions rapidly break down in the oral environment, leaving erosions (**181**) and ulcers (**182**).

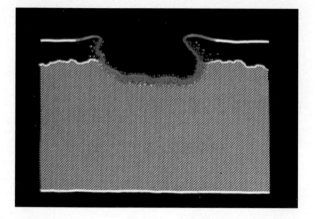

condition as being essentially bullous. There have been a number of reports linking oral bullous diseases (in particular, pemphigus or pemphigoid-like conditions and erythema multiforme) to internal malignancy in some patients, but the evidence for this is not entirely clear. The occasional occurrence of lesions of this kind in drug-induced conditions is, however, well established.

Pemphigus

Pemphigus (pemphigus vulgaris) is a potentially fatal bullous disease caused by acantholysis (loss of intercellular attachment) in the epithelium of both skin and mucosae (**183**). The floor of the resulting bullae is lined by the remaining basal cell layer, whilst the bulla fluid contains floating epithelial cells showing signs of acantholysis. These cells (Tzank cells) are a valuable diagnostic feature if bulla fluid can be obtained. Circulating autoantibodies to intercellular substances and structures can be detected and demonstrated (by immunofluorescence techniques), and then deposited around and between the epithelial cells of the stratum spinosum (**184**). This is the definitive diagnostic technique, invaluable in the differential diagnosis of the bullous diseases.

The skin lesions in pemphigus consist of bullae which may rupture rapidly (**185**) and from which the fragile epithelium may be lost to form eroded areas (**186**) which easily become infected. The earliest oral lesions may occur well before the onset of skin lesions—their bullous nature being difficult to identify since they almost immediately rupture, leaving eroded area of mucosa with rather ragged edges (**187**). Biopsy of an intact bulla may be impossible, but a specimen taken from intact mucosa adjacent to a ruptured bulla is likely to show the diagnostic immunofluorescent features. In more developed cases, the oral bullae may be large (**188**) and very fragile (**189** and **190**), the end result being widespread ulceration of the oral mucosa (**191**) with scarring and periodontal destruction as a long-term effect (**192**).

Pemphigus

Diagnosis: Cytology: Tzank cells in bulla fluid if available; biopsy of tissue adjacent to oral lesion. Immunofluorescence studies essential.

Important differential diagnosis: From other bullous diseases. Pemphigus is potentially fatal.

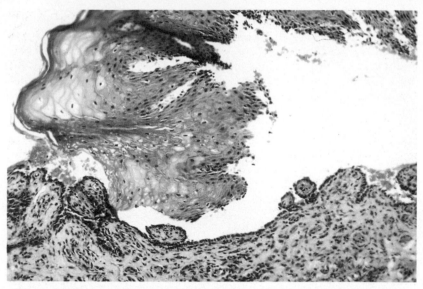

183 Pemphigus—histology showing the intra-epithelial split which is the cause of the lesions. The floor of the bulla is still lined by the basal cell layer of the epithelium.

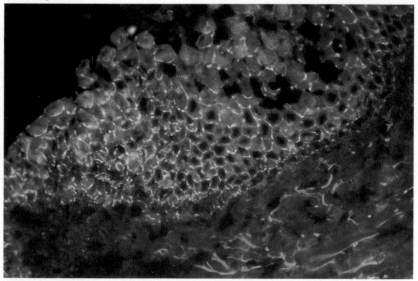

184 Pemphigus—autoantibody complexes lying around and between the cells of the stratum spinosum, demonstrated by immunofluorescent techniques.

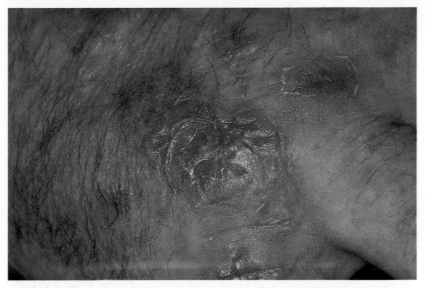

185 An early skin lesion in pemphigus—it is evidently a bullous lesion although the fluid has already been lost.

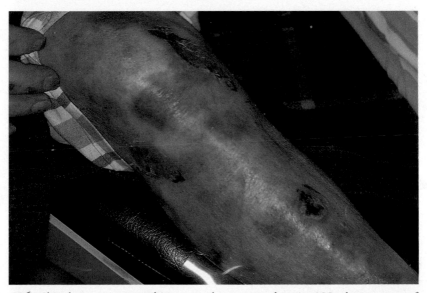

186 Skin lesions in pemphigus at a later stage than in **183**—large areas of epithelium have been lost.

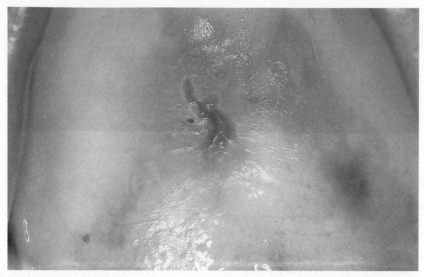

187 Early palatal lesions of pemphigus—these lesions were the earliest signs of the disease.

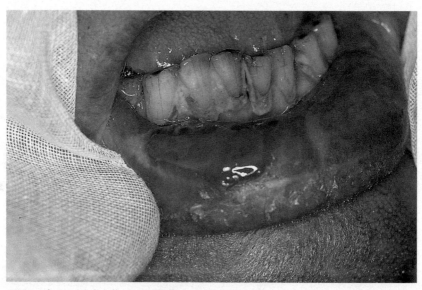

188 A large and still intact bulla of the lower lip in pemphigus—such bullae are very short lived.

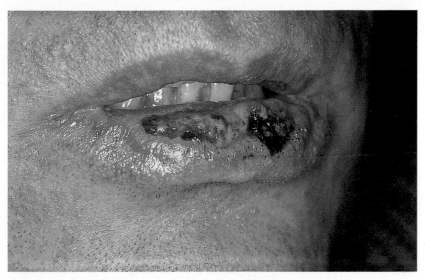

189 Ruptured bullae of the lower lip in pemphigus—a much more characteristic finding than the intact bullae shown in **186.**

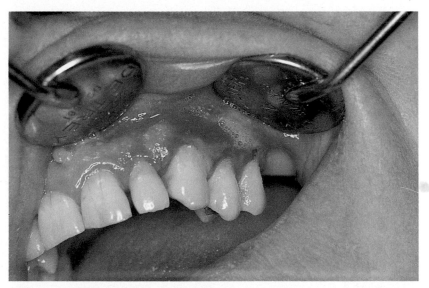

190 Erosive gingival lesions in pemphigus.

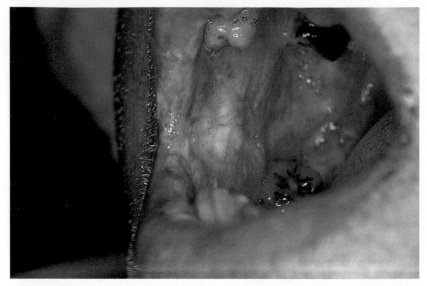

191 Pemphigus with widespread erosions of the buccal mucosa caused by the rupture of multiple bullae.

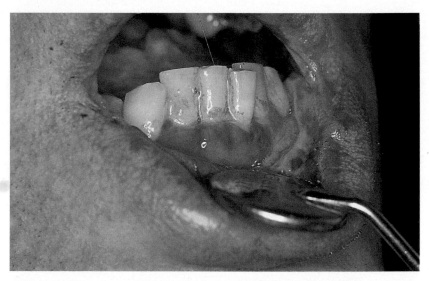

192 Pemphigus in a patient in which the skin lesions were under reasonable control—there is still instability of the oral mucosa, with scarring and severe periodontal loss.

Pemphigoid

Pemphigoid is a disease of the skin and mucosa of which there are a number of variants, in all of which sub-epithelial bullae are formed. There have been many classifications adopted, but there is little to be lost by using a simple division into two groups: generalised and mucosal pemphigoid. Generalised pemphigoid is a condition with bullae essentially of the skin, but sometimes with mucosal lesions. In mucosal pemphigoid, the predominant lesions are of mucous membranes, the skin being infrequently involved. The oral mucosa is almost always involved in mucosal pemphigoid and, often, the eyes.

Pemphigoid as it appears in the oral medicine clinic for diagnosis is almost always of the mucosal type—the oral bullae in generalised pemphigoid only rarely appear before the skin lesions. In all variants, the bullae are formed by the lifting off of the epithelium intact from the underlying connective tissue (**193**). Immunofluorescent techniques demonstrate immune complexes lying along the basal zone (**194**). The majority of patients with mucosal pemphigoid are between the ages of 50—70 at first presentation, and there is a preponderance of female patients (4:1 is the author's series). The bullae appearing on the oral mucosa are initially less fragile than those in pemphigus (**195**), but these eventually rupture, leaving eroded areas of mucosa (**196**). The gingivae are often involved, resulting in either erosive gingivitis (**197**) or, in less active cases, in a desquamative gingivitis difficult to distinguish clinically from that in lichen planus (**198**). In some patients, the pemphigoid bullae are relatively few in number, occur only infrequently and heal without scarring (**199**)—this has been described as intermittent mucosal pemphigoid.

A form of pemphigoid in which healing with scarring occurs is known as cicatricial pemphigoid (**200**). An older term—'benign mucous membrane pemphigoid'—has also come to be identified with this form of the disease. Although the scarring in the mouth—particularly seen in the palatal mucosa—gradually resolves, the equivalent process in the eye may lead to permanent damage. It is therefore necessary that all patients diagnosed as suffering from pemphigoid in any of its forms should have the benefit of an ophthalmic examination.

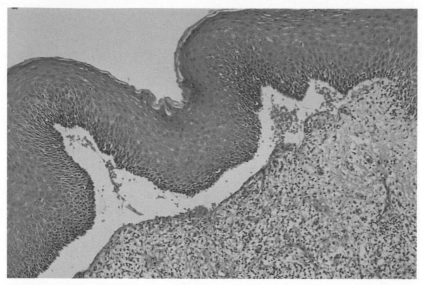

193 Pemphigoid—histology showing the epithelium (including the basal layer) lifted intact to form the bulla. Compare with **183.**

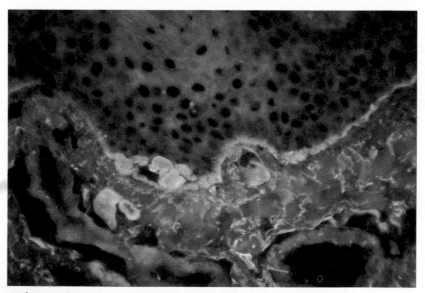

194 Pemphigoid—antibody complexes lying along the basal zone. Compare with **184**.

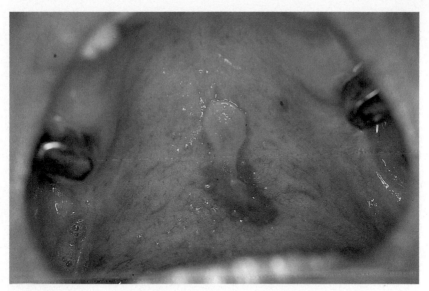

195 A ruptured palatal bulla in mucosal pemphigoid—the epithelium is still relatively intact.

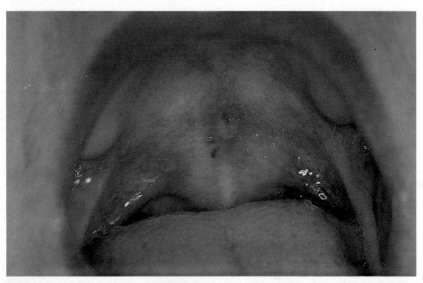

196 Typical palatal lesions in mucosal pemphigoid after rupture of the bullae.

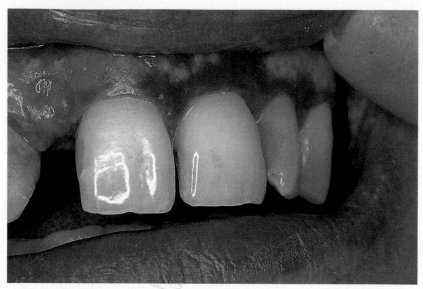

197 Erosive gingivitis in mucosal pemphigoid.

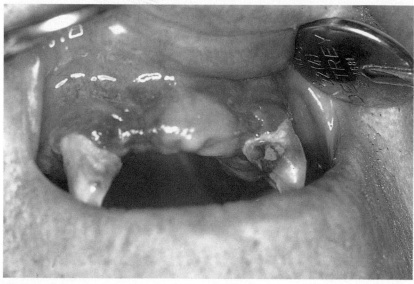

198 Desqumative gingivitis in pemphigoid— less erosive than in **197**.

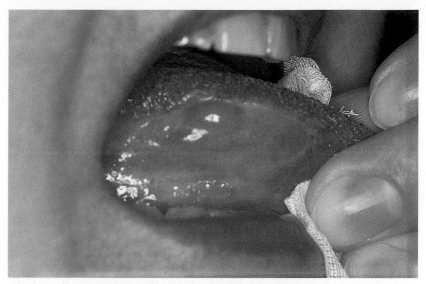

199 Pemphigoid—an intact bulla on the tongue. In this case, the bullae were few, and infrequent—intermittent mucosal pemphigoid.

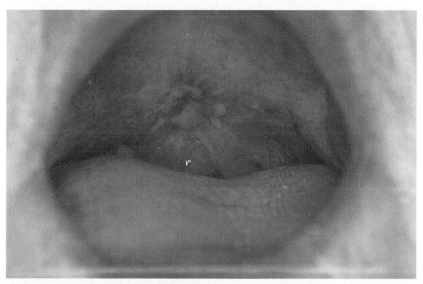

200 Scarring of the soft palate in cicatricial pemphigoid (benign mucous membrane pemphigoid).

141

Pemphigoid

Diagnosis: Biopsy; immunofluorescence studies essential.

Important differential diagnosis: From pemphigus. (The features of pemphigus and pemphigoid are summarised in **Table 14**, below.)

TABLE 14   Diagnostic Features in Oral Pemphigus and Pemphigoid

Pemphigus:
Fragile bullae—rapidly break down
Skin and mouth affected
Half of all cases begin in mouth
Patients predominantly 40-60 years
No sex preponderance
High incidence of Jewish patients
Rapidly progressive disease

Generalised pemphigoid:
Mouth involved in only 20% of patients
Few oral bullae
Bullae relatively firm
Most patients 60 years +
No sex preponderance
No ethnic prevalence
Less rapidly progressive than pemphigus

Mucosal pemphigoid: Mouth involved in virtually all patients
Skin lesions rare
Wide age range (30 years +)
Most patients 50 years +
Female preponderance (4:1)
No ethnic prevalence
Oral lesions may heal with scarring
Gingivae often involved

Also to be considered in differential diagnosis:
Bullous lichen planus
Idiopathic blood blisters

Erythema multiforme

Erythema multiforme is an acute bullous condition in which the oral mucosa (amongst others) may be involved together with the skin. It is possibly an immune complex disease, resulting from a wide range of antigens. In most cases, however, it is impossible to determine the precipitating factor for the condition. Most patients are young adults, and in many patients, the mouth and lips only are involved. There is a male preponderance of patients—in the order of 3:1. The more widespread version is known as the Stevens–Johnson syndrome, which may include widespread skin lesions and lesions affecting the eyes and genitals. Both the clinical and the histological features are variable, hence the term 'multiforme'

It is rare for oral bullae to be seen as such before their disintegration, the epithelial covering of the bullae being very fragile (**201**, **202**, **203** and **204**). The lips are particularly involved (**205**), which is a diagnostic feature. The oral lesions are accompanied by cervical lymphadenopathy, and there is a generalised malaise. The skin lesions (if they are present) are very characteristic (**206** and **207**). Numerous initiating factors, including drugs, have been recognised, some of which are given in **Table 13.** In many patients, the attacks are repeated in what becomes a recognisable pattern, although the reason for this may be elusive. If, however, a precipitating factor is recognised (for instance, recurrent herpes), then elimination or treatment of this may abort the next and subsequent attacks of the erythema multiforme. In a very few patients the episodes become prolonged and almost continuous. In even fewer patients the episodes are much less aggressive in nature, and the lesions are equally less troublesome (**208**), although repeated as in the more acute pattern.

201 Erythema multiforme—histology showing inter- and intra-epithelial cell oedema. There is also some sub-epithelial oedema. These features are very variable.

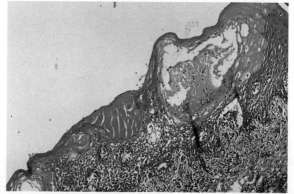

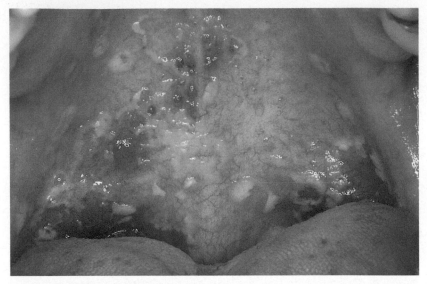

202 Erythema multiforme, at an early stage, affecting the palate. There are still remnants of ruptured bullae although most lesions have broken down to form erosions.

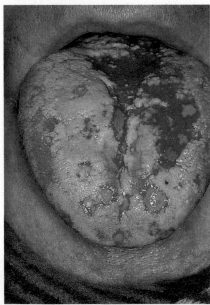

203 Erythema multiforme affecting the tongue. Ruptured bullae and heavy coating due to stasis and secondary infection. The presentation pictured is very similar to that in acute herpetic stomatitis (see Chapter 1).

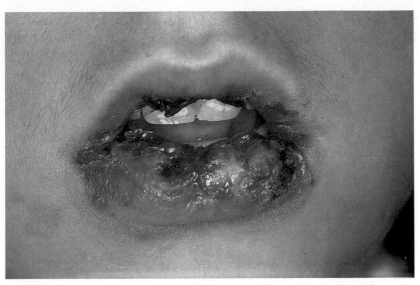

204 Lip lesions in erythema multiforme—a very characteristic feature.

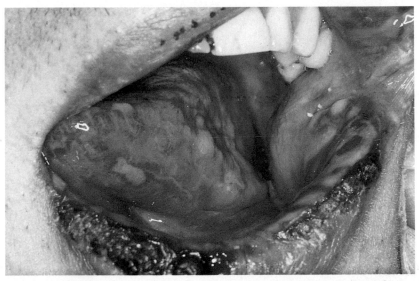

205 Widespread oral lesions of erythema multiforme, with crusting of the lips.

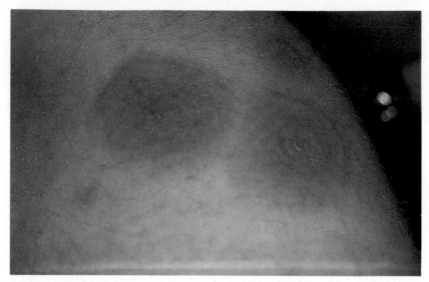

206 Target lesions of the skin in erythema multiforme.

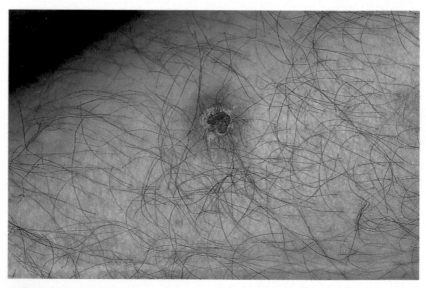

207 A target lesion of the skin in erythema multiforme with a central scab following rupture of a bulla.

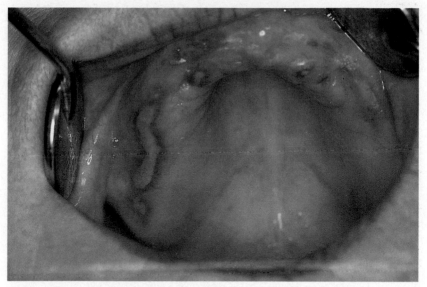

208 A less-aggressive variant of erythema multiforme affecting the alveolar mucosa.

Erythema multiforme

Diagnosis: Essentially clinical. Biopsy difficult to interpret. Associated lesions: 'target' lesions of skin, genital or eye inflammation.

Important differential diagnosis: From acute herpetic stomatitis. See **Table 15** (overleaf).

**TABLE 15   Acute Herpetic Stomatitis: Erythema Multiforme—
Clinical Features**

Acute herpetic stomatitis

One attack only
No previous history of herpes
Skin involvement—perioral only
No generalised lesions (eyes, genital etc.)
May be recent contact with herpes
Malaise
Cervical lymphadenopathy
Usually in young children, young adults
Male : female = 1 : 1

Erythema multiforme

Recurrent attacks common
May be previous history of herpes
May be precipitated by herpes
May be precipitated by drugs
Lip involvement characteristic
Skin lesions diagnostic when present
May involve eyes, genitals
Malaise
Cervical lymphadenopathy
Often in young adults; rarely in young
children
Male : female = 3 : 1

Epidermolysis bullosa

Epidermolysis bullosa is a term used to describe a group of closely
related, rare and genetically determined conditions affecting the skin
and mucosae—the type illustrated here is the dystrophic form in
which the abnormalities are gross. There is sub-epithelial blistering of
the skin and oral mucosa, leading to extreme fragility (**209** and **210**)
and to scar formation which restricts mouth opening. In addition
there is hypoplasia of the dental tissues (**211**). The overall result is
enormous problems of a dental nature—a reasonable standard of oral
hygiene is very difficult for the patient to attain, and dental treatment
is extremely difficult to carry out in view of the mucosal and skin
fragility and the restricted mouth opening.

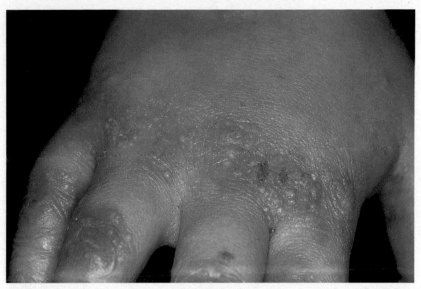

209 Skin lesions in epidermolysis bullosa showing multiple blister formation and skin fragility.

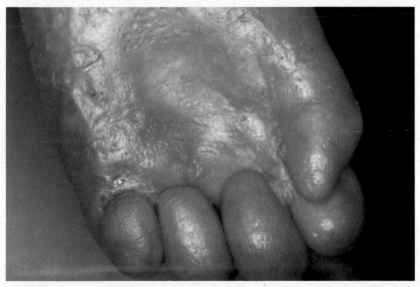

210 Gross tissue distortion with loss of fingernails due to repeated scarring lesions in epidermolysis bullosa—a severely affected patient.

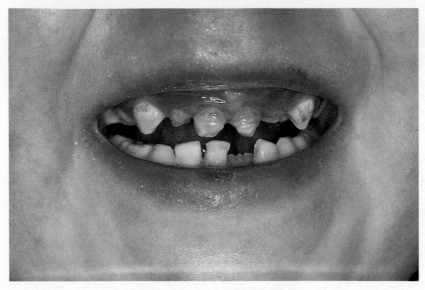

211 The teeth in epidermolysis bullosa showing hypoplasia. There is severe restriction in mouth opening due to repeated scarring.

Chapter 8

Connective Tissue Diseases, Sjogren's Syndrome and Xerostomia

Connective tissue diseases

The term 'connective tissue disease' (CTD) is used to describe a group of conditions, related by clinical and immunological similarities, in which connective tissue changes result from autoimmune processes. Although clearly defined conditions are well established, there is some degree of overlap of symptoms in this group—a fact emphasised by the condition known as 'mixed connective tissue disease', in which some of the characteristics of several of the diseases may be found in a single patient.

The designation 'connective tissue disease' is in some ways an unsatisfactory one in that a wide range of manifestations may occur which may not be directly attributable to changes in the connective tissues. However, it is an established term and its meaning is generally understood. An alternative designation is 'collagen vascular diseases'. In **Table 16** (overleaf), the diseases of this group are shown, together with their predominant clinical features.

There are two major oral factors of significance in relation to connective tissue diseases. The first is that mucosal lesions may occur in all but rheumatoid arthritis. Such oral lesions may appear early in the disease and therefore may be of considerable diagnostic significance. In some cases—particularly in systemic lupus erythematosus—the oral lesions may take the form of painful and intractable ulcers which present great problems of management. In other cases, the oral lesions may be relatively inactive and may clinically resemble those of lichen planus. The second significant factor is that any of these diseases may be associated with salivary gland hypofunction and consequent xerostomia as part of secondary Sjogren's Syndrome (SS)—discussed below. The oral manifestations of CTD are summarised in **Table 17** (page 159).

Rheumatoid arthritis

There are no specific oral mucosal changes in rheumatoid arthritis (RA), the most common of the connective tissue diseases. However, temporomandibular joint (TMJ) is affected in a significant proportion of patients with RA—grossly so in some acute cases. Problems of mal-

TABLE 16 Connective Tissue Diseases—Predominant Clinical Features[*]

Rheumatoid Arthritis (RA)	Arthropathy
Systemic Lupus Erythematosus (SLE)	Skin rashes (often photo-sensitive) Renal diease (variable type) Lung involvement Cardiomyopathy Neurological changes Arthropathy Vasculitis Raynaud's phenomenon
Chronic Discoid Lupus Erythematosus (CDLE)	Skin rashes Mucosal lesions
Systemic Sclerosis (Scleroderma) (SSc)	Fibrosing skin and mucosal lesions GI tract lesions Vasculitis Reynaud's phenomenon Pulmonary fibrosis Cardiomyopathy Renal disease leading to: Hypertension
Polymyositis (Dermatomyositis)	Myositis Skin rashes

There may be some overlap of features in all these conditions.

occlusion may follow—in particular, an 'open bite' caused by the erosion of the condyle heads. The symptoms are of pain and tenderness in the TMJs, with difficulty in movement. On stethoscopic examination, loud crepitus may be heard. Radiography may show rheumatoid changes in the TMJs similar to those in other joints (**212** and **213**). Severe TMJ disturbance is, however, relatively rare. In most cases, the joint changes and consequent symptoms are relatively mild and only slowly progressive—often there are periods of activity followed by resting phases.

RA is often associated with Sjogren's syndrome—it has been reported that at least 50% of all patients diagnosed as having RA also have some degree of xerostomia.

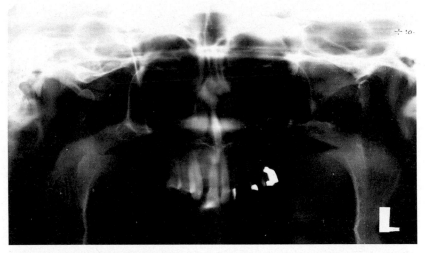

212 Radiograph showing arthritic changes in the temporomandibular condyle heads and fossae in rheumatoid arthritis.

Rheumatoid arthritis

Diagnosis: First diagnosis of RA on oral signs/symptoms alone very unlikely. Immunological tests for RA. Radiography (TMJ).

Differential diagnosis: Other conditions causing polyarthropathy, e.g. psoriatic arthropathy, TMJ/muscle dysfunction syndrome.

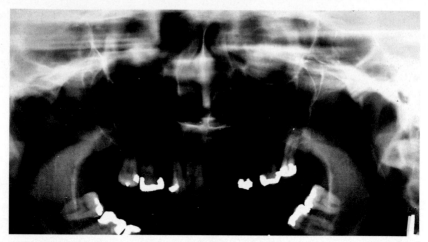

213 Major destruction of the condyles in uncontrolled severe and acute rheumatoid arthritis. As a result, the patient had a marked anterior open bite.

Systemic lupus erythematosus

Systemic lupus erythematosus (SLE) is a generalised autoimmune condition with a broad spectrum of activity—there may be widespread changes in the connective tissues, with secondary effects on the cardiovascular and respiratory systems, renal tissues and skin, amongst others. The joints, including the TMJs, may be affected. SLE may be a slowly progressive condition or may, in some patients, take a rapid, aggressive and potentially fatal course. The majority of patients with the acute form of the disease are females, aged 10–40 years. Skin involvement is a common feature, often accompanied by widespread and painful oral ulceration (**214**). The skin rashes may be precipitated by exposure to sunlight. Generalised symptoms include malaise, pyrexia and loss of weight. SLE may occur as a drug-induced condition—there have been many drugs implicated, including those responsible for lichenoid reactions and erythema multiforme (see Chapter 7). The predominant oral manifestation is the ulceration mentioned above; secondary Sjogren's syndrome occurs in 30% of patients. The diagnosis is made by the recognition of the characteristic immune abnormalities—almost all patients have circulating antinuclear antibodies (ANA) (**215**). In many patients, LE cells may be recognised—these are immunologically modified leukocytes formed by incubation of the patients' own polymorphs and serum, which includes the specific LE factor.

154

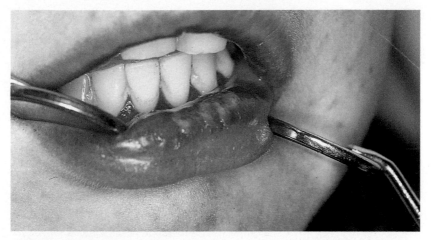

214 Painful ulceration of the lower lip in a fifteen-year-old female patient with systemic lupus erythematosus.

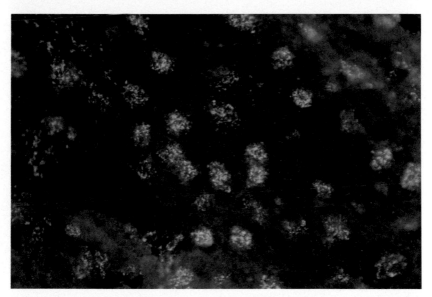

215 Antinuclear antibodies demonstrated by immunoflourescent techniques in a patient with SLE. Until recently, such antibodies were described by their distribution in the target nuclei (this is the speckled type) but much more site-specific immunological tests are rapidly becoming available—those specified for the investigation of Sjogren's syndrome are examples.

Systemic lupus erythematosus

Diagnosis: Immunological tests. In a few cases, oral biopsy with immunofluorescence may be difficult to interpret.

Chronic discoid lupus erythematosus

Chronic discoid lupus (CDLE) is a much more restricted form of lupus than SLE, largely affecting the skin and causing relatively few systemic abnormalities. The skin rash is often facial, with a butterfly distribution across the bridge of the nose, and may be accompanied by oral or lip lesions which may have a resemblance to lichen planus (**216** and **217**). The skin rash is often photosensitive. As in SLE, there is a preponderance of female patients. The immunological findings are much less positive than in SLE.

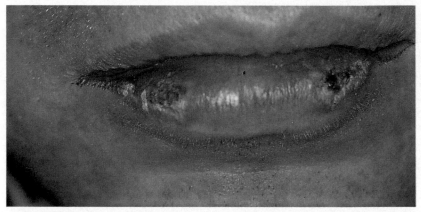

216 Crusted lesions of the lower lip in chronic discoid lupus. These are the most common oral manifestation of CDL.

Chronic discoid lupus erythematosus

Diagnosis: Immunological tests variable. Biopsy may be difficult to interpret.

Important differential diagnosis: From oral lichen planus.

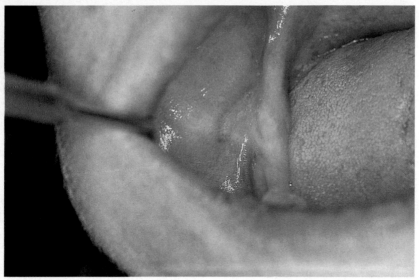

217 A faint white lesion of the buccal mucosa in a patient with chronic discoid lupus. This—the only lesion apart from a facial rash—was found to have the histological features of CDL on biopsy.

Systemic Sclerosis (Scleroderma)

The essential change in systemic sclerosis (SSc) is the laying down of dense fibrous tissue in the dermis of the skin and mucous membranes, and also in other organs (lungs and heart). There may be any one of a number of renal changes, which may lead in turn to secondary hypertension. Vasculitic changes and Raynaud's phenomenon also occur. The skin and mucosal changes may show up markedly in the face, with the lips and cheeks becoming inflexible and wrinkled, reducing the ability to open the mouth (**218**). The tongue may become immobilised, and mastication may be difficult. There are no characteristic oral mucosal lesions described in SSc, but a radiographic widening of the periodontal ligament has been described—particularly in relation to the posterior teeth.

Systemic Sclerosis (Scleroderma)

Diagnosis: Clinical. Immunological tests are non-specific.

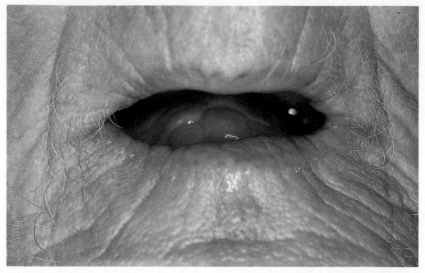

218 Scleroderma—restriction in the flexibility of the facial tissues and in mouth opening.

Polymyositis (Dermatomyositis)

In polymyositis and its variant, dermatomyositis, there is a generalised myositis with progressive muscular weakness. There may or may not be an associated skin rash. Although oral mucosal lesions have been described in a few patients, these have been inconsistent in nature, and no characteristic oral lesion has been identified.

Mixed Connective Tissue Disease (MCTD)

In this overlap condition, the patient may have a combination of the features usually associated with more than one connective tissue disease. This combination may occur simultaneously or in sequence. The clinical features include Raynaud's phenomenon, polyarthralgia, myositis, skin rashes and any of the features described in other CTD. The orofacial manifestations include trigeminal neuropathy leading to neuralgia-like pain or partial or complete anaesthesia, cervical lymphadenopathy and xerostomia. A case has been reported in which an oral mucosal lesion occurred, resembling lichen planus clinically but

TABLE 17 Connective Tissue Diseases—Predominant Oral Features

Rheumatoid Arthritis (RA)

TM Joint Involvement

Systemic Lupus Erythematosus (SLE)

Oral ulceration

Chronic Discoid Lupus Erythematosus (CDLE)

Keratotic mucosal lesions

Systemic Sclerosis (SSc)

Restriction of mouth opening

Mixed Connective Tissue Disease (MCTD)

Trigeminal neuropathy

---

* *All may be associated with xerostomia as part of Sjogren's syndrome.*

not histologically (**219** and **220**). Patients have a high level of a specific antibody to RNase-sensitive extractable nuclear ribonucleoprotein (RNP) antigen—this is diagnostic. Antinuclear antibodies (speckled type) are positive.

Mixed Connective Tissue Disease (MCTD)

Diagnosis: Immunological.

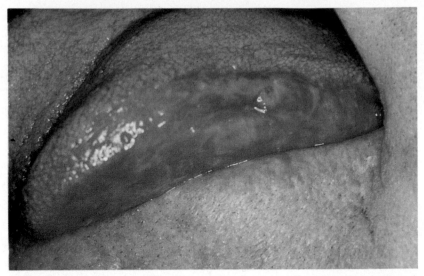

219 A lesion of the lateral margin of the tongue at first thought on clinical grounds to be of lichen planus. Biopsy showed, however, a different picture (**220**).

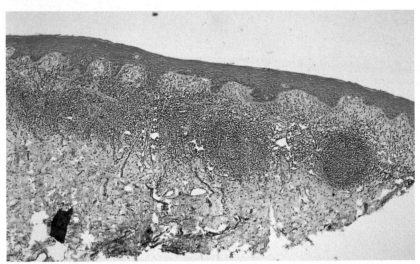

220 The histological appearance of the lesion shown in **219** with focal aggregates of lymphocytes not typical of lichen planus. The eventual diagnosis was of mixed connective tissue disease. This is a very rare combination of circumstances but illustrates the value of biopsy as a confirmatory procedure.

Xerostomia

It has long been assumed that increasing age results in loss of salivary gland function in the normal individual with resultant xerostomia (dry mouth). However, all recent work in the field implies that this is not so and that in healthy, non-medicated individuals, salivary function may continue with only minimal reduction due to increasing age. The clinical assessment of xerostomia is notoriously difficult and carefully controlled salivary flow rate tests are required to objectively establish the diagnosis. Some of the common causes of xerostomia are shown in **Table 18**. Xerostomia as a side effect of therapeutic drugs is probably the most common contemporary cause of the complaint of dry mouth.

TABLE 18 Xerostomia: Common Causes

Sjogrens' Syndrome	Primary
	Secondary
Psychogenic	(Including depression)
Drug-induced	Antidepressants
	Tranquillizers
	Antihypertensives
	Antihistamines
	Many others
Diabetes mellitus	
Less common causes	Neurological disease
	AIDS
	Post-radiation involving glands

Xerostomia

Diagnosis: If felt necessary, as for the salivary component of Sjogren's syndrome (below).

Sialorrhoea

The reverse condition, excessive salivation (sialorrhoea), is comparatively rare. It may be complained of by patients wearing new dentures, and represents a response to a foreign body in the mouth. Ulcerative or infective lesions of the mouth (including neoplasms) may also lead to a stimulated salivary flow. In a very few patients (predominantly those with myasthenia gravis under treatment with anticholinesterases), excess salivation may be a side effect of drug therapy. In a significant number of patients, complaints of intermittent excessive salivary flow may accompany conditions such as the burning mouth syndrome as a stress-related, non-physically demonstrable condition.

Sjogren's Syndrome

Sjogren's syndrome (SS) is an autoimmune condition affecting the secretory function of the salivary and lachrymal glands and leading to the symptoms of dry mouth and dry eyes. It is most commonly associated with one of the connective tissue diseases, in which case it is known as secondary SS. In the absence of such an association, the term 'primary SS' is now used—the previously used term was 'Sicca Syndrome'. Specific autoantibodies have now been identified as being present in SS.

As a result of the xerostomia, the mouth becomes dry—often distressingly so—with burning and other subjective symptoms ('cracking', 'splitting' etc). The oral mucosa may be erythematous, and the tongue often loses its normal surface structure (**221**). Taste sensation may be distorted, and cervical caries may be a considerable problem (**223**). Secondary candidiasis may occur, including angular cheilitis (**222**). There may be swelling of the major salivary glands (**224**), but this is by no means constant. Very rarely, non-neoplastic gross swelling of the palatal minor salivary glands may also occur (**225**). Due to the lack of tear secretion, the eyes feel irritable, with a 'foreign body' sensation and possible photophobia (**226**). Secondary changes in SS include sialadenitis and calculus formation as a result of the hypofunction of the salivary glands (**227**).

In SS, the normal architecture of the salivary glands is lost, with atrophy of the secretory units and a lymphocytic infiltration of the stroma. These changes occur in the major salivary glands and also in the minor salivary glands distributed around the oral mucosa, including the mucosa of the lips. This is the basis of the labial gland biopsy procedure, which is an important diagnostic test in the definitive diag-

221 The dry tongue of a patient with Sjogren's syndrome associated with SLE. In other patients depapillation may be more prominent and a careful assessment must be made to eliminate secondary haematological changes such as those shown in Chapters 3 and 4.

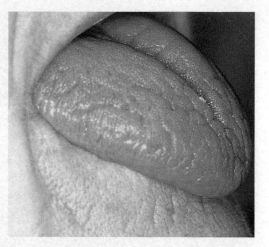

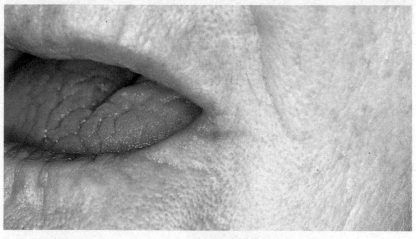

222 Angular cheilitis in Sjogren's syndrome. The organism involved was *Candida albicans*.

nosis of SS (**228**). The function of the major salivary glands may be determined by nuclear medical methods similar to those used to investigate thyroid function—the scintiscan technique (**229, 230, 231** and **232**). The scintiscan gives much more information about the function of the salivary glands than do contrast radiographs, which predominantly demonstrate structural changes (**233**).

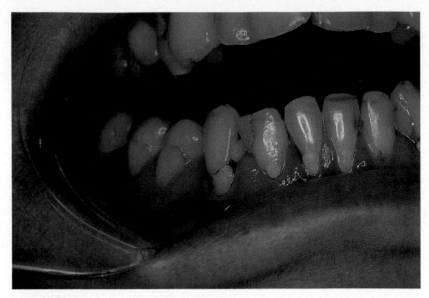

223 The typical picture of a patient with long-standing xerostomia due to SS. The lack of appreciation of the likelihood of rapid cervical caries has led to multiple restorations.

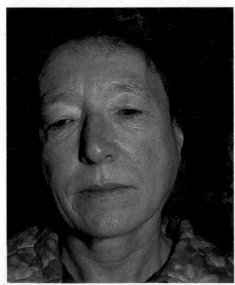

224 Parotid swelling in Sjogren's syndrome.

225 Swelling of the palatal minor salivary glands in Sjogren's synrome—a much less common finding than that of parotid swelling.

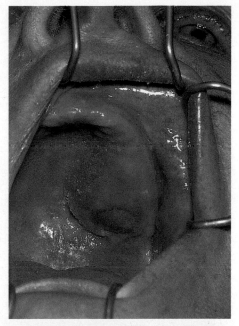

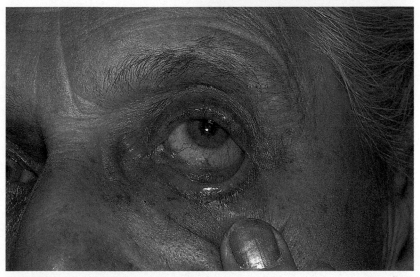

226 A keratoconjunctivitis resulting from the reduced tear secretion in Sjogren's syndrome.

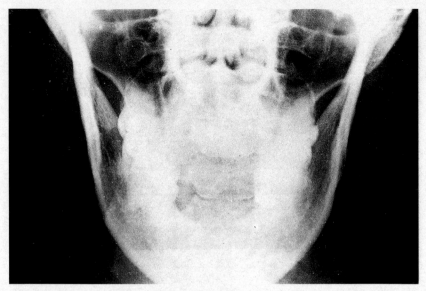

227 Multiple small parotid calculi following reduced secretory activity in Sjogren's syndrome.

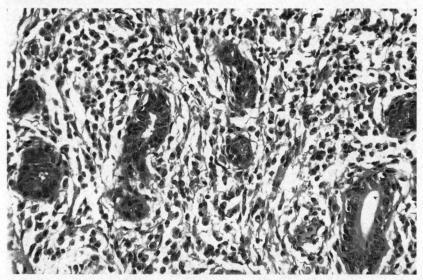

228 Section from the biopsy of a labial minor salivary gland in Sjogren's syndrome. There is loss of secretory units, hyperplasia of the ductal epithelium and lymphocytic infiltration.

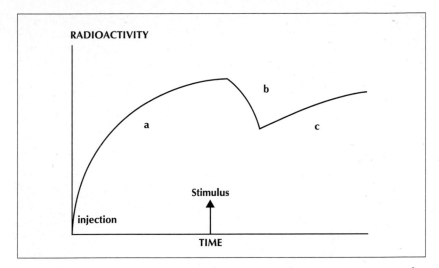

229 Diagrammatic representation of computerised time-activity curve of a normal salivary gland during scintiscanning. An intravenous injection of radioactive labelled pertechnate is given—part 'a' of the curve represents the uptake of this by the gland. At 'stimulus', usually after ten minutes, lemon juice is introduced into the mouth and part 'b' of the curve shows the 'washing out' effect. Following this the uptake continues slowly to increase to a maximum and then slowly decline ('c').

230 An actual print-out of the time-activity curves for the four major salivary glands in a normal patient. Each colour represents the output from one gland.

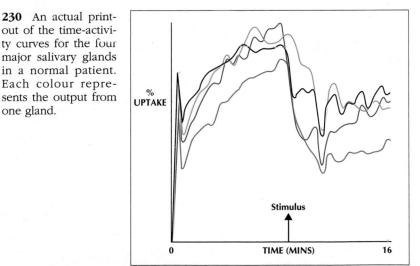

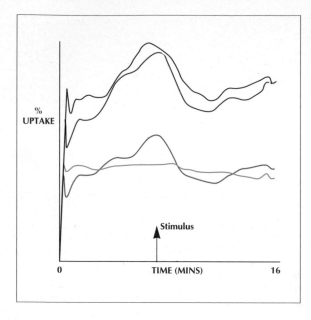

231 In this printout, one gland (right submandibular—green) is virtually non-functional. The others show a normal response.

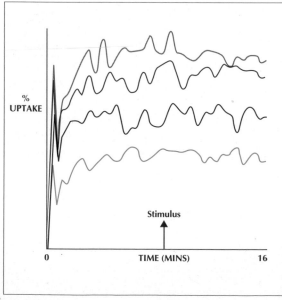

232 In this scintiscan, all four major salivary glands show poor uptake and poor response to the stimulus—findings consistent with Sjogren's syndrome.

Sjogren's syndrome

Diagnosis: Salivary flow rate tests (very difficult to carry out on an individual basis), Scintiscan to determine gland function. Representative sialogram to determine major structural changes in gland. Immunology (presence of SSA/Ro, SSB/La). Labial gland biopsy. All patients should have an expert ophthalmological examination.

Sialosis

Sialosis is a relatively uncommon non-inflammatory and non-neoplastic condition affecting the major salivary glands, causing swelling and occasional pain. The causes of this condition are multifactorial—some are shown in **Table 19**. Histologically, there is proliferation of secretory units with atrophy of the ducts—the mechanisms are not understood. In those patients with a recognisable causative factor, the process may be reversed by taking appropriate steps to deal with this.

TABLE 19   Sialosis: Associated Conditions*

Nutritional and related	Anorexia
	Alcoholism
	General malnutrition
	Malabsorption
Generalised diseases	Diabetes mellitus
	Liver cirrhosis
	Endocrine disturbances
Drugs implicated	Propanalol
	Isoprenaline
	Methyldopa
	Iodine
	Phenylbutazone

This is not a complete list—other conditions and drugs have been implicated with varying degrees of evidence.

Sialadenitis

Inflammatory changes in the salivary glands are most commonly acute and are the result of viral infections, of which mumps is by far the most common. The mumps virus is directly transmitted and primarily affects the major salivary glands—in particular, the parotids. It is almost always diagnosed by its clinical features, although immunological tests are available and, should the facilities be available, the mumps virus is at once identifiable on electron microscopy of the saliva.

Bacterial sialadenitis (acute or chronic) is most commonly a secondary condition, following duct obstruction or degenerative changes in the salivary glands (as in Sjogren's syndrome). An acute infection, ascending from the mouth, may occur in some patients who are in poor general health. This was once a common sequel to surgery, but is now virtually never seen in this context. Chronic bacterial sialadenitis—particularly of the parotids—may follow the primary changes of degenerative salivary gland disease, or be the eventual result of stasis following duct obstruction caused, for instance, by a calculus (**233**). Very occasionally, essentially chronic infections (such as tuberculosis or actinomycosis) may involve a salivary gland.

Sialadenitis

Diagnosis: Clinical, reinforced by microbiological tests. Causes of swelling of the major salivary glands are summarised in **Table 20**. An important cause for confusion in the case of the parotid gland is an inaccurate appreciation of its anatomy. Abnormal bulk of the masseter muscle (as demonstrated in masseteric hypertrophy) is often misdiagnosed as parotid swelling (**234**).

TABLE 20 Salivary Gland Swellings—Often Most Prominent in the Parotids

Chronic	Sjogrens' syndrome
	Sialosis
	Neoplasia (usually unilateral)
	Sarcoid
	AIDS
	Infections (eg Tuberculosis)
Acute	Viral sialadenitis (eg Mumps)
	Bacterial sialadenitis (usually secondary)
	Acute obstruction
	Allergy (rare)

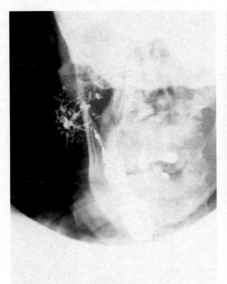

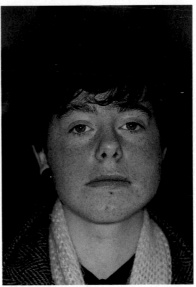

233 Contrast sialogram of the right parotid gland of the patient with the scintiscan shown in **232** (page 168). The report was 'consistent with autoimmune sialadenitis with superimposed chronic obstructive sialadenitis'.

234 Right-sided masseteric hypertrophy—often mistaken for parotid swelling.

Necrotizing sialometaplasia

This is a rare condition, but one which may cause a disproportionate degree of alarm since it is often mistaken, on both clinical and histological grounds, for a malignant neoplasm. Changes of an unknown nature—but probably vasculitic—affect groups of minor salivary glands in the palatal mucosa. There is breakdown of the overlying mucosa with the production of an apparently aggressive ulcer (**235**). Biopsy may show pseudoepitheliomatous hyperplasia of the overlying epithelium, which may easily be interpreted as indicating malignancy. However, this is in fact a self-limiting and self-healing condition.

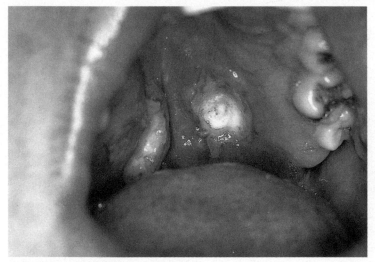

235 Palatal ulceration in necrotizing sialometaplasia.

Chapter 9

Immflammatory Overgrowths, Vascular Lesions and Related Conditions

Inflammatory overgrowths

Inflammatory overgrowths of the oral mucosa, including the gingivae, are common. By and large, these lesions are clinically recognisable, and fall into well-defined groups. The most usual cause of such lesions of the mucosa in general (but not of the gingivae) is chronic mechanical trauma.

Fibro-epithelial polyp: Denture granuloma

The fibro-epithelial polyp consists essentially of scar tissue produced as a response to trauma. Its most common site is on the buccal mucosa, in relation to the occlusal plane (**236**), but other locations may be involved (**237** and **238**). The lesions are characteristically pedunculated. These lesions are generally regarded as entirely benign. When a fibro-epithelial polyp occurs under the fitting surface of an upper denture, it may assume a disc-like form which is compressed into a depression in the palatal mucosa (**239**). The pedicle is developed into a small hinge from which the flap-like lesion may be displaced downwards (**240**). These instantly recognisable lesions are given a variety of names, including 'leaf fibroma' and 'palatal papilloma'. Neither of these indicates the true nature of the lesion. The 'denture granuloma' is a similar lesion to the fibro-epithelial polyp, modified by the local tissue morphology and the nature of the irritant—the flange of a denture (**241** and **242**). There are many variants in the name used to describe this common condition ('denture-induced hyperplasia', etc.).

Fibro-epithelial polyp

Diagnosis: Almost entirely clinical; the features are very characteristic.

Important differential diagnosis: As in all other cases of tissue overgrowths, from neoplasia.

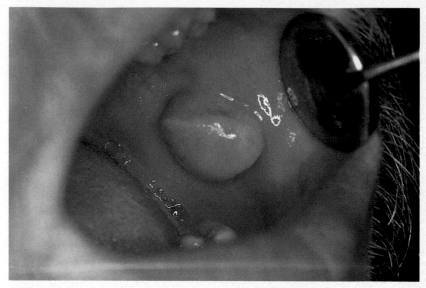

236 A quite typical, although large, fibro-epithelial polyp on the buccal mucosa. The continuing trauma which has been responsible for its growth is demonstrated by the faint white keratotic line on the occlusal plane.

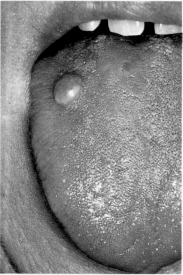

237 A fibro-epithelial polyp in a less common site—the dorsum of the tongue.

238 A fibro-epithe-lial polyp of the palate in an edentu-lous patient. This lesion was quite asymptomatic and the patient was able to accommodate to its slow growth.

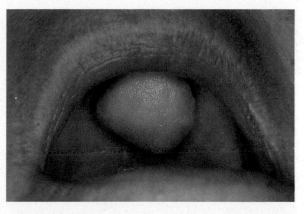

239 A palatal polyp in a patient wearing a full upper den-ture—the polyp is compressed into a shallow recess in the palatal mucosa.

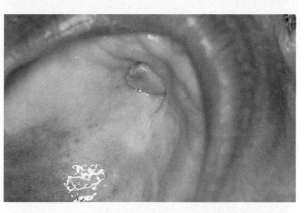

240 A polyp such as that shown in **239** displaced downwards on the hinge formed by the pedicle.

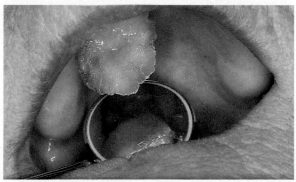

175

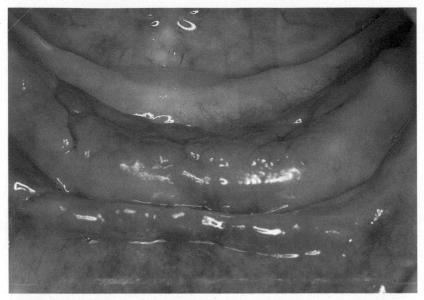

241 A denture granuloma in the lower buccal sulcus—its linear form represents the area irritated by the denture flange.

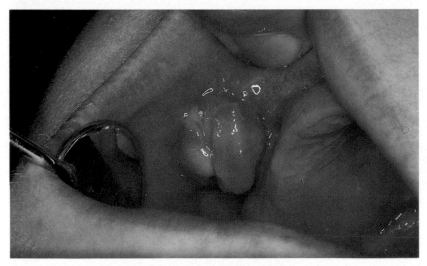

242 A less typical denture granuloma—the irritation has been localised to a restricted area of the buccal mucosa. None the less, the fissured structure of the lesion, caused by the friction of the denture flange, is evident.

Epulis

The term epulis (plural: epulides) has the literal meaning of a swelling on the gum. It is used to describe a range of discrete lesions produced as a result of inflammatory changes at the gingival margin. It has no specific histological connotations, although there are generally recognised groups within the spectrum of inflammatory changes seen in these lesions. The fibrous epulis, essentially consisting of mature granulation tissue, grows slowly and often causes the patient little trouble (**243**). Its precise colour and texture depend on the degree of maturity of the lesion and on the presence or absence of secondary inflammatory changes. For some obscure reason, there seems to be a preponderance of female patients with a fibrous epulis, although the quoted figures vary widely (from 2 : 1 to 4 : 1). Neglect of the relatively symptom-free lesion may lead to the eventual production of unusually large epulides (**244**). These are often traumatised and hence, secondarily ulcerated. There seems to be very little, if any, premalignant potential in these lesions, but it must always be remembered that, very occasionally, true neoplasms (either primary or secondary) may appear at the gingival margin.

Immature forms of the fibrous epulis may appear in which the granulation tissue remains vascular and immature, with a higher cellular content and lower fibrous content than the more usual fibrous epulis (**245**). The rather ill-defined term 'pyogenic granuloma' is often used to describe these lesions, although it is a term also used in other clinical contexts. Occasionally, lesions with a similar histological appearance occur in non-gingival sites (**246**). Epulides with this immature structure have the reputation of being more difficult to eliminate by simple excision than do the more mature fibrous variety. Vascular epulides often appear as part of the 'pregnancy gingivitis' picture (see Chapter 11).

In the giant cell epulis (**247**), there is an osteogenic component, and the tissue includes a variable number of multinucleated giant cells. Depending on the maturity of the lesion, bone formation may occur. There are wide discrepancies in the reported figures relating to the age and sex of the patients. Very occasionally, a lesion histologically resembling a giant cell epulis may arise in the soft tissues adjacent to an edentulous alveolus (**248**). It has been suggested that, in a very few patients, a giant cell epulis may be a manifestation of hyperparathyroidism, although the characteristic giant cell lesion in this condition is intrabony.

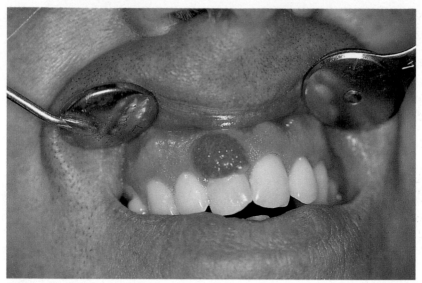

243 A simple fibrous epulis.

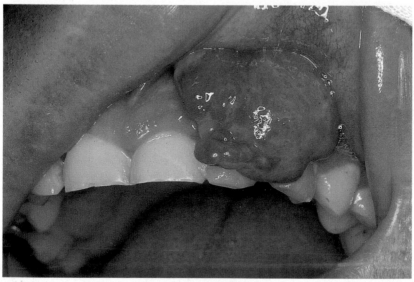

244 A large and long standing fibrous epulis with some degree of secondary ulceration due to trauma. There are no reported cases of malignant change in such lesions—however large they may grow.

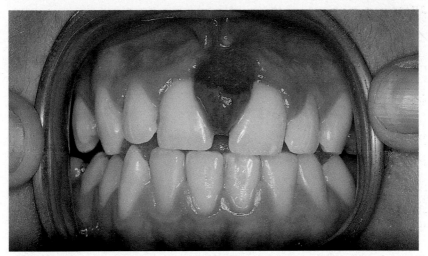

245 This is an immature vascular epulis (the so-called pyogenic granuloma type). There are no particular clinical features to distinguish these from the more fibrous types, although they tend to be more apparently vascular and fragile, leading to bleeding on contact.

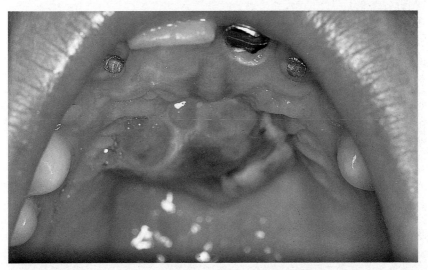

246 A palatal polyp with a rather immature structure similar to the vascular epulis.

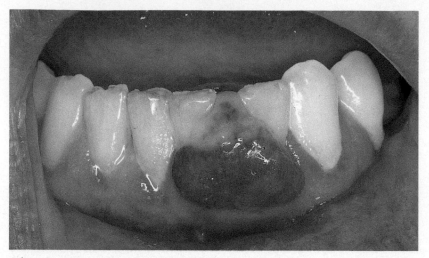

247 A giant cell epulis. Again there is no definitive clinical appearance although the giant cell variants are reputed to have a rather purple appearance compared to the fibrous types.

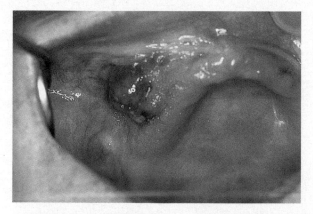

248 A giant cell epulis in the mucosa adjacent to the edentulous alveolus.

Epulis

Diagnosis: Clinical, confirmed by histology. Consider the necessity for screening for hyperparathyroidism in giant cell epulis.

Important differential diagnosis: From primary or secondary neoplasm.

Papilloma

A papilloma is not an inflammatory overgrowth but a true benign epithelial neoplasm with (in the oral cavity) virtually no tendency to malignant change. These lesions are relatively common, and may occur in almost any site in the mouth (**249**). The most frequent site, however, is at the junction of the hard and soft palate (**250**). The 'cauliflower-like' appearance of the lesions is very characteristic, and is almost diagnostic. (The role of the papilloma virus has been mentioned in Chapter 1.) Viral warts—common on the hands and fingers of children—may be transmitted to the oral mucosa and lips by biting or chewing these lesions (**251** and **252**). Although unsightly, viral warts have a limited life and may be expected to regress spontaneously.

249 A papilloma on the ventral surface of the tongue.

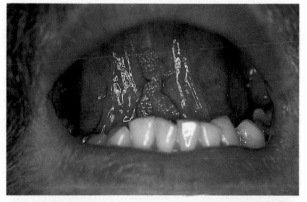

250 A palatal papilloma in a characteristic site. As often occurs, there is evident secondary trauma from the back margin of the denture. The 'cauliflower'-like structure is quite characteristic of a papilloma rather than of a fibro-epithelial polyp.

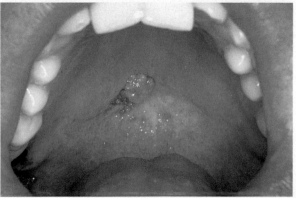

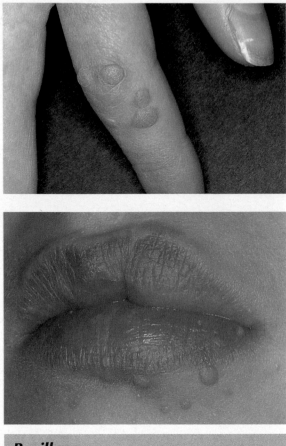

251, 252 Viral warts transmitted from the fingers to the lips.

Mucous cyst

Mucous cysts (mucoceles) are small cysts arising from the mucous glands of the oral mucosa and are usually the result of trauma—the lower lip is most commonly affected (**253**). The blue and translucent appearance is very characteristic. In some cases, after the initial traumatic incident, the cystic lesion may burst and refill over a period of time. Occasionally, mucous cysts may arise in sites in which a traumatic origin is less demonstrable (**254** and **255**).

253 A typical small mucous cyst of the lower lip.

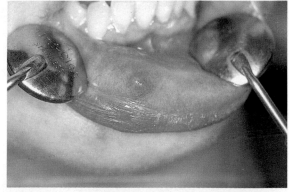

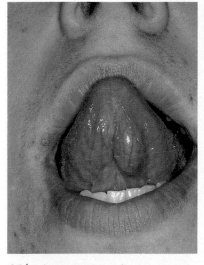

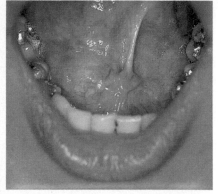

254 A mucous cyst in an uncommon site—the ventral surface of the tongue.

255 A mucous cyst lying in the floor of the mouth is known as a ranula—in a few cases it may be derived from the major sublingual salivary gland and be a much less superficial structure than it appears.

Mucous cyst

Diagnosis: Clinical.

Important differential diagnosis: From haemangioma.

Vascular lesions

Varicosities

Sublingual varicosities (**256**) may be considered a normal finding. Their increase as a simple age-related factor is unproven, but their prominence in patients with hypertension and peripheral vessel incompetence is generally accepted (**257**). These lesions may also be present on the buccal or labial mucosa (**258**).

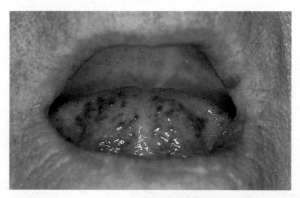

256 Normal sublingual varicosities in a middle-aged patient.

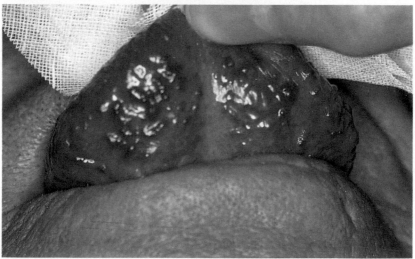

257 Exaggerated sublingual varicosities in a patient with cardiovascular disease. It is not clear how reliable a diagnostic indicator this is.

258 Buccal and labial varicosities in the patient shown in **257**.

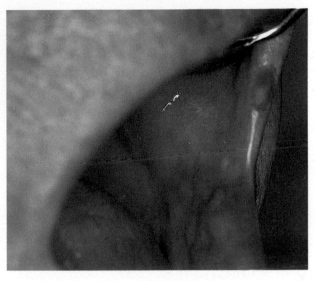

Hereditary haemorrhagic telangiectasia

In hereditary haemorrhagic telangectasia (Osler–Weber–Rendu syndrome), small areas of dilated and thin-walled blood vessels appear on the skin and mucous membranes (**259** and **260**). The oral mucosa is almost always involved, often as the first sign of the condition. Haemorrhage due to rupture of the abnormal vessels in the nasal mucosa often occurs, leading to epistaxis—oral bleeding is less common. Compare with the petechial haemorrhages shown in **121** and **123** (see Chapter 4).

Hereditary haemorrhagic telangiectasia

Diagnosis: Clinical, including family history. Telangiectic vessels blanch on pressure below a glass slide—petechial haemorrhages do not.

Important differential diagnosis: From petechial haemorrhages, as in thrombocytopenia (see above).

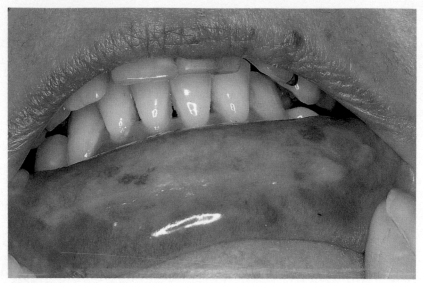

259 Small areas of dilated capillaries in the labial mucosa of a patient with hereditary haemorrhagic telangiectasia.

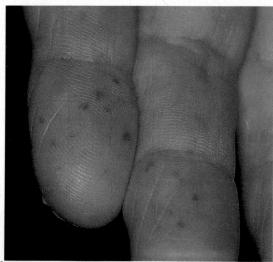

260 Skin lesions in the patient shown in **260.**

Haemangioma

Haemangiomas have been variously regarded either as benign neoplasms or as hamartomas. The usual criteria for neoplastic growth do not apply, since changes in haemodynamics are known to affect the size of haemangiomas. Oral haemangiomas most commonly affect the lips and tongue. Some are effectively static lesions (**261**), whilst others (**262**) may be rapidly expansile and pose great problems of management. It should always be established in lesions such as that shown in **262** that there is no involvement of the adjacent bone (**263**).

Haemangioma

Diagnosis: Clinical. Haemangiomas blanch on pressure. Imaging procedures may be necessary if bone involvement is suspected.

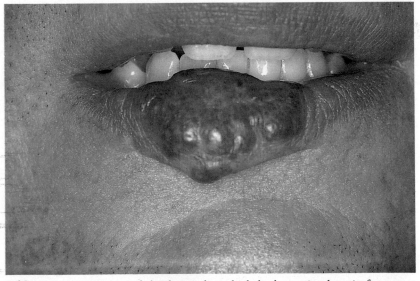

261 A haemangioma of the lower lip which had remained static for many years.

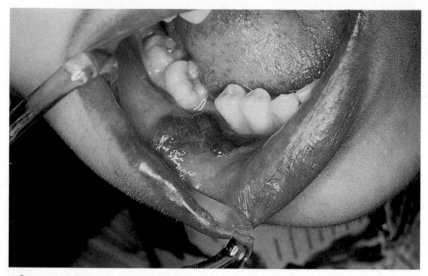

262 A rapidly expanding haemangioma involving the lower lip.

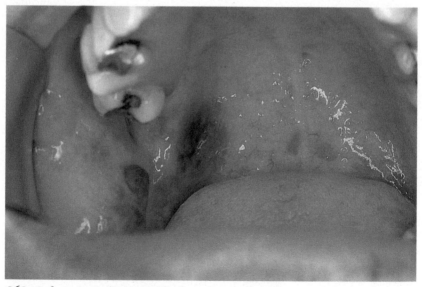

263 Soft tissue indications of a haemangioma with major bone involvement in the mandible and maxilla.

Chapter 10

Leukoplakia, Neoplasms and Related Conditions

Leukoplakia

The term 'leukoplakia' (white patch) is an entirely descriptive one and was used in the past to include a wide range of white lesions of the oral mucosa. It is currently used in the sense first defined by Pindborg and now generally accepted as 'a white patch on the oral mucosa which cannot be wiped off and which is not susceptible to any other clinical diagnosis'. In this way, a range of white lesions (such as those of lichen planus and pseudomembranous candidiasis) are excluded from this precise definition.

Leukoplakia has long been considered an essentially premalignant condition. However, with the adoption of the above definition, which contains no element of prognosis or of histological implications, this interpretation can no longer be accepted. The term 'leukoplakia' remains an entirely clinical one and is generally accepted as implying a lesion of non-specific histology, with a variable behaviour pattern but with an unpredictable (but statistically assessable) tendency to malignant transformation. In an individual case, the most reliable indicator of potentially malignant behaviour is the assessment of representative biopsy material by an expert observer. This remains largely a subjective process in spite of many efforts to introduce more objective criteria.

Some lesions have been considered to be related to leukoplakia and also to be, to some extent, its precursors. 'Leukoedema' is the term used to describe a condition in which the oral mucosa and, in particular, the buccal mucosa, present with a translucent whitish-grey appearance, rather as if a superficial film were lying on the surface of the mucosa (**264**). This film of rather oedematous epithelial cells may be at least partly scraped off. Opinions vary about this condition—some consider it to be a normal finding, whilst others associate it with tobacco smoking. Racial differences have been described, and there is no doubt that the condition may be much more apparent in patients with deeply pigmented mucosae. One reason for the great variability in the reported incidence of leukoedema in different surveys may

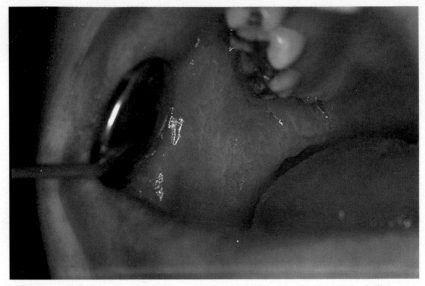

264 Asymptomatic leukoedema in a patient smoking 30 cigarettes daily.

well be the difficulty in visualisation under artificial light sources as distinct from natural light. The term 'pre-leukoplakia' has been used by a number of epidemiological investigators to describe an intermediate stage in the formation of leukoplakia. The lesion is diffuse and white, being less dense and less marked than one which would merit the term 'leukoplakia' (**265**). The implication is that more well-defined lesions which would merit the term 'leukoplakia' are likely to appear. The histological changes in pre-leukoplakia are likely to be much less well defined than in the more fully developed lesions.

A leukoplakia may appear at any site on the oral mucosa. Its subsequent behaviour and, most importantly, its potential for malignant transformation cannot be predicted with complete accuracy. However, both the site and the clinical features are known to affect prognosis, whilst the histological features shown on biopsy are of great importance in attempting to assess future behaviour. Homogenous leukoplakias of the kind shown in **266** are least likely to show epithelial atypia on biopsy and, even in quite heavy tobacco smokers, may show limited epithelial atypia (**267**). The floor of the mouth and the ventral surface of the tongue are common sites for leukoplakia, often forming the so-called 'ebbing tide' pattern (**268**). It was for some time thought that these characteristic lesions were of

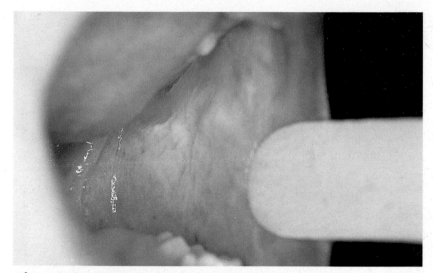

265 Preleukoplakia in a 13-year-old male with a genetically determined tendency to oral leukoplakia associated with oesophageal carcinoma and tylosis. (See also **287** and **288**.)

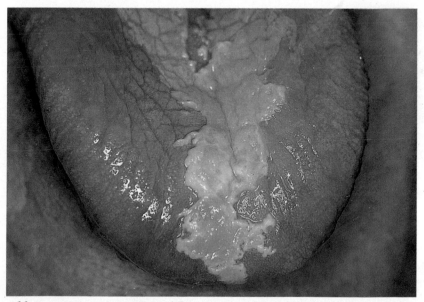

266 Homogenous leukoplakia of the dorsum of the tongue in a male, aged 83.

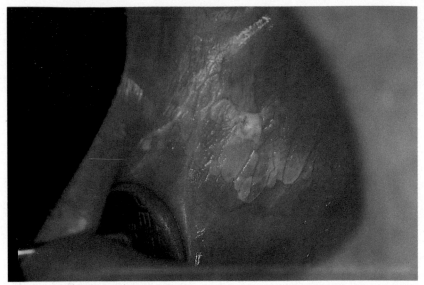

267 Homogenous leukoplakia of buccal mucosa and commisure. Although the patient smoked 50 cigarettes daily, there were few signs of epithelial atypia on biopsy.

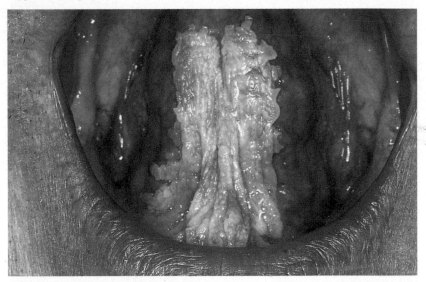

268 Leukoplakia of the floor of mouth and ventral surface of the tongue showing the so-called 'ebbing tide' pattern.

very low premalignant potential and possibly of developmental origin, but it is now quite clear that their behaviour is as unpredictable as those in other sites. Figures based on retrospective surveys imply that the potential for malignant transformation in this site is in fact greater than in most other oral sites (**269**). In particular, the onset of red atrophic patches in the lesion (erythroplakia) (**270**) should be taken as an early warning indicator of potential malignancy. In speckled leukoplakia, white areas alternate with areas of atrophic red epithelium (**271**)—the site illustrated (at the commisure) is quite characteristic, although other sites may be involved. These lesions are frequently associated with candidal infiltration, and have a considerably higher incidence of malignant transformation than do homogenous leukoplakias. All leukoplakias with a recognisable candidal infiltration of the epithelium on biopsy (**272**) and those presenting clinically with associated areas of erythroplakia must be treated with suspicion as having a relatively high chance of undergoing malignant change. Although the precise role of the candida is unknown and its function as a precipitating agent or as a secondary infective agent is undecided, there are many clinical situations in which leukoplakia seems to develop in pre-existing areas of angular cheilitis (**273**). The extension of an angular leukoplakia distally from the commisure to involve the

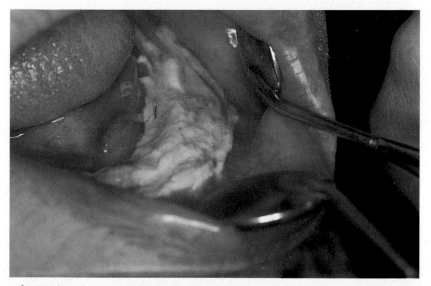

269 Widespread leukoplakia of alveolar mucosa and floor of mouth showing marked epithelial atypia on biopsy.

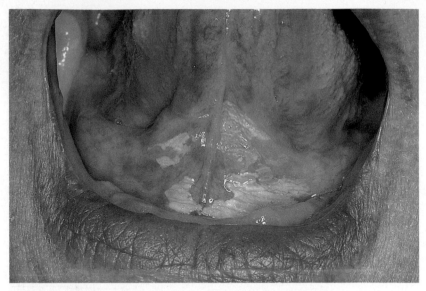

270 Leukoplakia of floor of mouth with areas of erythroplakia.

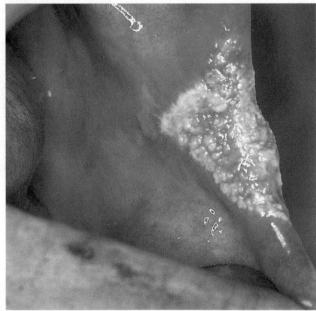

271 Speckled leukoplakia of the commisure —characteristic in site and in appearance.

272 A section from a biopsy of a leuko-plakia, stained with periodic acid—Schiff reagent (PAS), show-ing candidal pseudo-hyphae penetrating the outer layers of the epithelium—can-dida leukoplakia or chronic hyperplastic candidiasis.

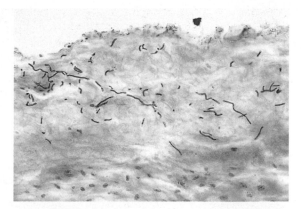

273 An early candi-dal leukoplakia developing in an area of long-standing angular cheilitis.

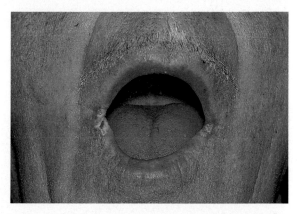

buccal mucosa is common (**274**). Candidal leukoplakia as the clinical manifestation of chronic hyperplastic candidiasis has been discussed in Chapter 1.

Syphilitic leukoplakia of the tongue has also been mentioned in Chapter 1. Although a classic manifestation of the later stages of the disease, it is now rarely seen in European conditions. The characteris-tic picture is of diffuse leukoplakia and erythroplakia of the tongue, often with marked epithelial atypia on biopsy and with a very high malignant potential (**275**). It is suggested that this condition is a mani-festation of secondary immunodeficiency consequent on the primary syphilitic infection.

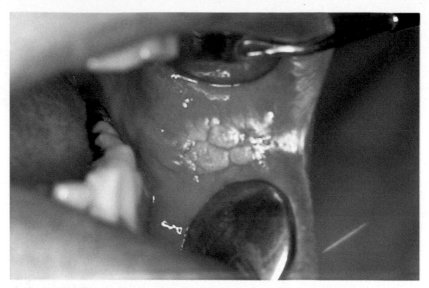

274 Candida leukoplakia of the buccal mucosa and commissure.

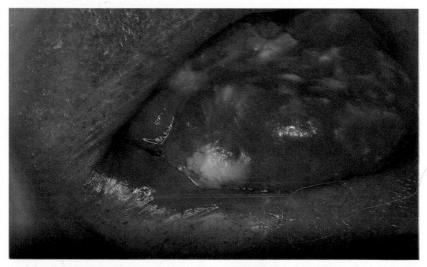

275 Leukoplakia of the tongue, with associated erythroplakia, in a patient with late inadequately treated syphilis.

The tendency of the lower lip to be subject to potentially malignant lesions been outlined in Chapter 3, and the role of sunlight as an aetiological factor was mentioned. Occasionally, a quite different type of lesion may occur—more hyperplastic and hyperkeratotic than the rather atrophic 'lip at risk' lesion (**276**). It is not clear whether such lesions also share the high malignant potential of the atrophic lesions.

The effect of trauma in the production of leukoplakia is minor. Simple frictional keratoses are common (**277** and **278**), but it has not been demonstrated that these are precursors of lesions showing significant epithelial atypia. Similarly, the common lesion resulting from a cheek-chewing habit (**279**) is considered to be entirely without premalignant implications.

276 Leukoplakia of the lower lip with minimal epithelial atypia on biopsy.

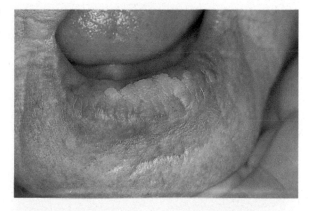

277 Frictional keratosis of the buccal mucosa resulting from a traumatic denture.

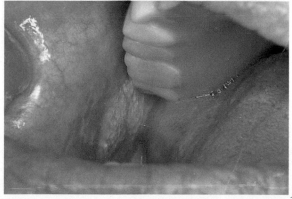

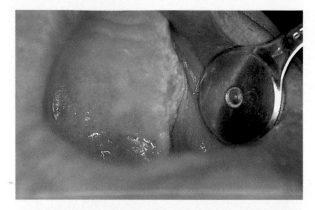

278 Frictional keratosis of the edentulous alveolar ridge mucosa caused by long-term mastication without dentures.

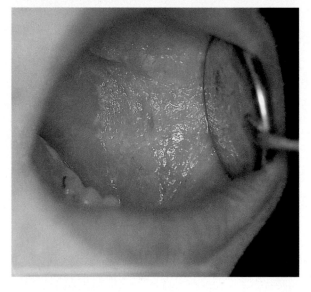

279 A typical lesion caused by a cheek-chewing habit, with small eroded areas and loose tags of partially detached mucosa.

The role of tobacco in the aetiology of leukoplakia is well established. Tobacco smoking and chewing habits have been repeatedly shown to increase considerably the incidence of leukoplakia in the groups studied. In general the incidence of epithelial atypia in tobacco-related lesions is high, although somewhat unpredictable in individual cases—as in the lesion shown in **267**. In general, tobacco-related lesions may be expected to regress on reduction or cessation of the habit, but there are reported instances in which this has proved to be a transient effect (**280**, **281** and **282**). The effect of tobacco usage in patients with concurrently existing abnormalities of the mucosa (such as lichen planus) is generally to intensify the degree of epithelial abnormality found on biopsy (**283**).

A quite specific tobacco-related lesion is the so-called 'smoker's keratosis' of the palate. In the European environment this has been most frequently described in pipe smokers (hence the term 'pipe smokers' palate'), although almost any tobacco-smoking habit may be involved. The characteristic feature is the enlargement of the palatal mucous glands and the dilatation of their ducts to produce a central red spot. These stand out in contrast to the generally white background of the palatal mucosa and the palatal gingivae (**284**). This condition, perhaps rather surprisingly, seems to have virtually no potential for malignant transformation. The clinical features are so characteristic that it is generally considered that biopsy is not normally necessary for diagnosis. A palatal condition which shows some similarities to the smoker' s keratosis, but without the evident involvement of the mucous glands, is papillary hyperplasia (palatal papillomatosis). In this condition (which does not seem to be tobacco-related), a number of small papillomatous projections are present on the palatal mucosa (**285**). There have been widely divergent views as to the aetiology and the significance of this condition—the general current view is that it is entirely benign.

Leukoplakia

Diagnosis: Virtually all leukoplakias/erythroplakias should be biopsied. Clinical diagnosis is acceptable in a few cases, e.g. smoker's palatal keratosis or cheek chewing.

Important differential diagnosis: Leukoplakia/erythroplakia from lichen planus.

Most important differential diagnosis: All of the above conditions from carcinoma.

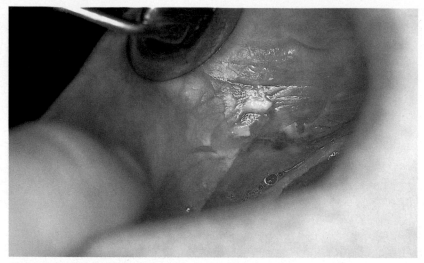

280 A buccal leukoplakia with areas of erythroplakia in a heavy cigarette smoker (50 daily). There were marked epithelial atypia and candidal infiltration on biopsy. Discontinuation of the smoking habit and antifungal therapy resulted in clinical regression of the lesion (see **281**).

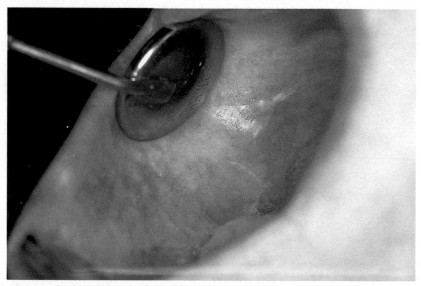

281 Marked regression of the lesion shown in **281** after three months without the use of tobacco. (See also **282**.)

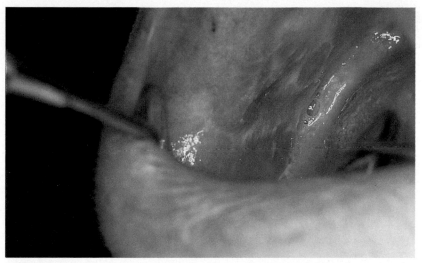

282 Partial recurrence of the lesion shown in **280** and **281** after one year without tobacco.

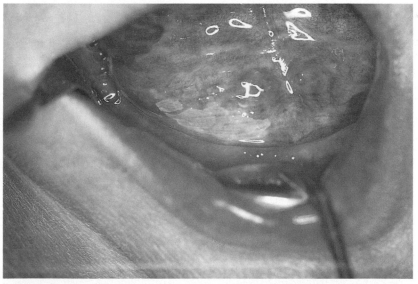

283 A lesion with the characteristics of lichen planus but with marked epithelial atypia on biopsy—the patient was a heavy cigarette smoker.

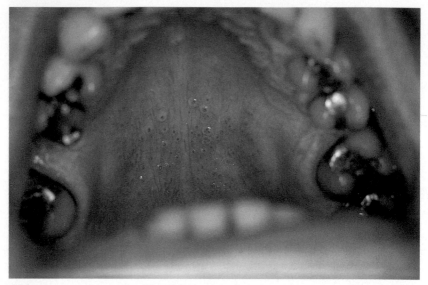

284 Smoker's keratosis of the palate. The involvement of the mucous glands helps to give the characteristic appearance.

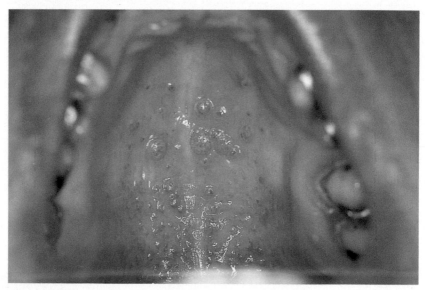

285 Papillary hyperplasia of the palate.

Developmental keratoses

Leukokeratosis or 'white sponge naevus' (there are many synonyms) is a hereditary disorder of keratinisation which affects all mucosae but, in particular, the oral mucosa (**286**). Generally, the diffuse lesions appear in childhood or early adolescence—they are quite symptomless, have no pre-malignant potential and the genetic mechanism is unclear.

There are a very few patients in whom disorders of keratinisation of the oral mucosa are accompanied by abnormalities of the skin or other mucosae (**287** and **288**). In this familial condition, hyperkeratosis of the palms and feet (tylosis) is associated with leukoplakia of the oral mucosa (pre-leukoplakia in childhood) and carcinoma of the oesophagus. This is a genetically dominant pattern. In other patients with tylosis unassociated with oesophageal carcinoma, simple keratotic lesions of the gingivae are not unusual (**289**). A number of such rare associations involving the skin and the oral mucosa have been described.

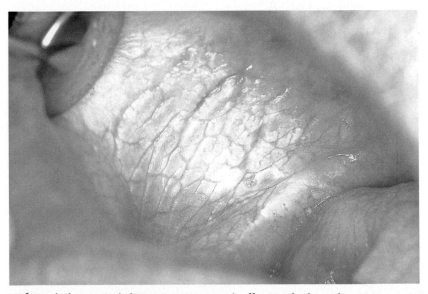

286 Leukokeratosis (white sponge naevus) affecting the buccal mucosa.

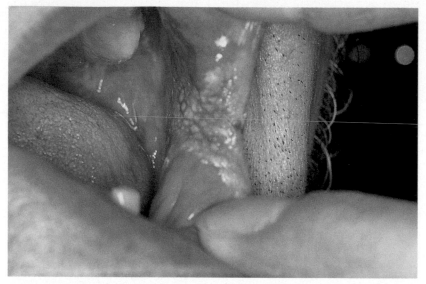

287 A leukoplakia of the commissure and buccal mucosa in a patient from a family with genetically linked tylosis and oesophageal carcinoma.

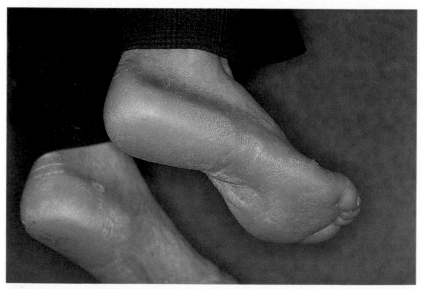

288 The feet of the patient shown in **288**—there is gross hyperkeratosis (tylosis).

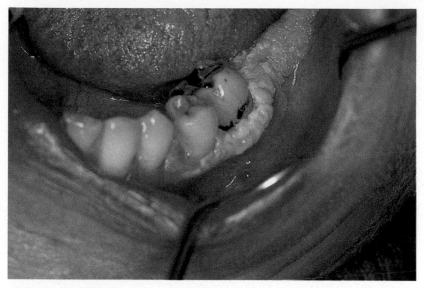

289 Gingival keratosis in a patient with tylosis not linked to oesophageal carcinoma.

Developmental keratoses

Diagnosis: Clinical and from the family history. If in doubt, biopsy.

Important clinical factor: To recognise the existence of complex conditions indicated by oral keratotic abnormality.

Submucous fibrosis

Submucous fibrosis (SMF) is a condition which occurs predominantly amongst inhabitants of the Indian subcontinent, Malaysia and nearby countries, although increasing numbers of patients have more recently been described from outside these areas. Dense fibrous tissue is laid down in the oral and pharyngeal submucosa, leading to stiffening of the tissues, binding down of the tongue and difficulty in mouth opening and in swallowing (**290**). There are subsequent atrophic changes in the oral epithelium which may transiently result in oral ulceration or vesicle formation, but which eventually cause the oral

205

mucosa to take on a marbled appearance (**291**). The oropharynx may also be involved. This is considered to be condition with a high potential for malignant change. The incidences of leukoplakia with epithelial dysplasia and of frank carcinoma have been shown to be very high in a number of surveys of patients with SMF. In spite of a great deal of speculation regarding food hypersensitivity and the role of tobacco and betel nut chewing habits, the cause of SMF remains undecided. Recent work has concentrated on genetic factors, in particular the HLA mechanism.

Fordyce's spots

This condition is included in this chapter, although it represents a completely normal situation. Fordyce's spots are the sebaceous glands of the oral mucosa, which vary considerably from patient to patient in number, distribution and prominence (**292**). During episodes of mild stomatitis (as, for instance, during the course of the common cold), the glands may appear more prominent than normal. Their greatest significance, however, is the fact that they are frequently mistaken for pathological structures and so are of importance in differential diagnosis.

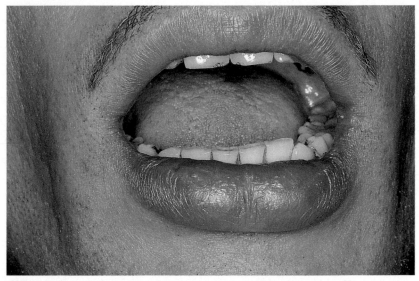

290 Restriction of mouth opening in a patient with submucous fibrosis.

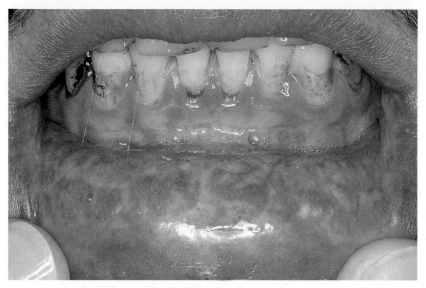

291 The marbled appearance of the labial mucosa in the patient with sub-mucous fibrosis shown in **290**.

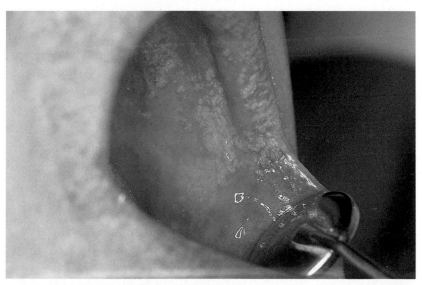

292 Fordyce's spots—the name given to the appearance of quite normal but prominent buccal sebaceous glands in some patients.

Carcinoma and other neoplasms

A wide variety of neoplasms, both benign and malignant, primary and secondary, may appear in the oral cavity. Of these, oral carcinoma is by far the most significant in terms of numbers and world-wide distribution. There is great variation in the incidence of oral carcinoma in various parts of the world, ranging from less than 5% of all cancers in Europe to over 30% in some Asiatic countries. In all parts of the world, however, oral carcinoma is a highly significant cause of morbidity and mortality. Metastatic growth may occur early—often in the presence of apparently insignificant primary lesions. Aetiological factors have been very intensively investigated; of these, tobacco smoking and chewing habits are by far the highest on the list of those implicated. High alcohol consumption in itself has not been shown to influence the incidence of oral carcinoma, but seems to have a synergystic effect when coupled with a tobacco habit. Other aetiological factors clearly depend on the precise site—such as the role of sunlight in inducing malignant change in the epithelium of the lips, as discussed in Chapter 3. Pre-malignant lesions have been discussed in the first part of this chapter, however it should be realised that by no means are all oral carcinomas preceded by a recognisable pre-malignant phase. Many start with no such recognisable warning sign. It should also be recognised that the aetiological factors for oral carcinoma may not be identical with those for leukoplakia.

Carcinoma

Oral carcinoma may present as a change in a pre-existing leukoplakia/erythroplakia (**293**) or as a new lesion, either proliferative (**294**) or ulcerated (**295** and **296**). In other cases, the lesion may present as a red or red and white patch, which might be clinically diagnosed as lichen planus or erythroplakia (**297**). In some cases, there are widespread changes over virtually the whole of the oral mucosa (**298**); in such circumstances it is difficult to determine whether this represents the transformation of a pre-existing leukoplakia or whether the lesion has arisen initially over the whole field. The possibilities of field change or multifocal lesions should always be considered when carrying out pre-treatment assessment in oral carcinoma. The importance of carrying out full clinical investigations in presumed carcinoma is shown in the case illustrated in **299**, in which a simple inflammatory lesion showed many of the superficial characteristics of a carcinoma of the floor of the mouth such as that shown in **300**.

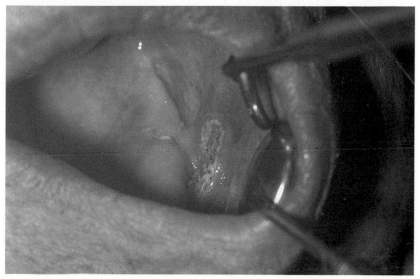

293 An early, quite symptom-free, carcinoma arising in the site of a previously excised leukoplakia.

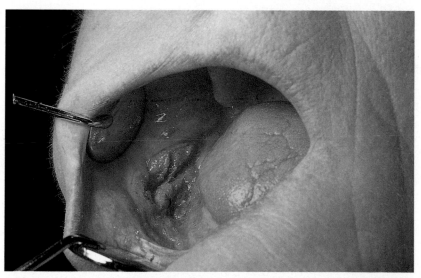

294 A carcinoma of the alveolar mucosa extending on to the buccal mucosa and floor of mouth. In this case there was minimal ulceration, and the lesion had been mistaken for a denture granuloma.

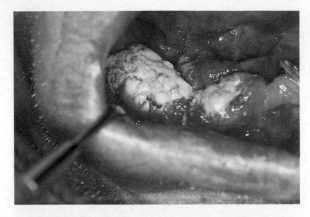

295 Advanced carcinoma of the alveolar mucosa, with gross ulceration and advanced bone destruction. The cervical lymph nodes were heavily involved.

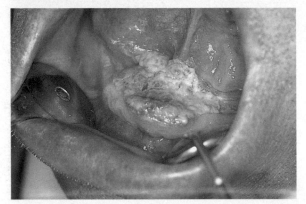

296 Carcinoma of anterior floor of mouth with widespread ulceration.

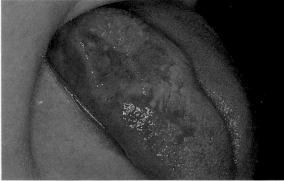

297 Carcinoma of the lateral margin of the tongue, presenting as an erythematous patch.

298 Widespread carcinoma of the oral mucosa. Virtually the whole of the mucosa was involved. In some areas the histology was of carcinoma, in others of candida leukoplakia with marked atypia.

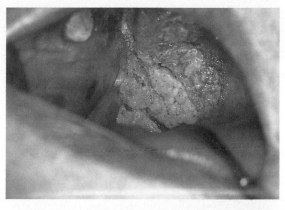

299 A secondarily traumatised and infected denture granuloma simulating a carcinoma—compare with **300**

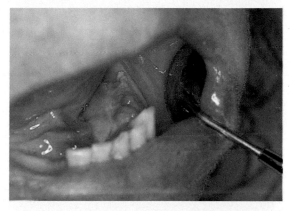

300 Carcinoma of floor of mouth—compare with the lesion shown in **299**.

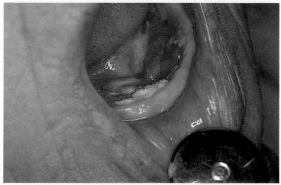

Carcinoma of the lip shows special characteristics which are not fully understood. The great majority of such carcinomas are in males and affect the lower lip (**301**). They are characteristically painless and slow growing, often being mistaken for a long-standing herpetic lesion. Metastatic spread generally occurs very late, and primary lesions may reach an appreciable size without the involvement of the cervical nodes which would be likely to occur in such long-standing lesions in other oral sites (**302**). Such carcinomas rarely have a precursor lesion and seem to represent a different disease pattern to the diffuse carcinomatous change which may occur in the 'lip at risk' (**303**)—see also Chapter 3.

The term 'carcinoma' has been used in this chapter as being synonymous with 'squamous cell carcinoma'. Basal cell carcinomas of the oral cavity are virtually unknown, apart from direct extensions from skin lesions, but occasionally an intra-oral lesion occurs with the structure of a verrucous carcinoma (**304**). These are generally regarded as being tobacco related.

Carcinoma

Diagnosis: Initially clinical recognition—a high degree of clinical suspicion is essential. Biopsy confirmation. Full clinical assessment, including possibility of multifocal primary lesions and metastatic spread. Imaging techniques (CAT scanning, magnetic resonance) may be helpful in delineating advanced lesions.

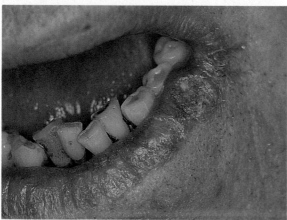

301 A small carcinoma of the lower lip of an older male patient. Characteristically, this had been mistaken for a particularly long-lasting herpetic lesion.

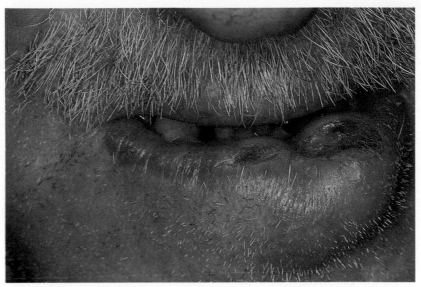

302 A long-standing and very slowly growing carcinoma of the lower lip. Even at this stage, there was no detectable lymph node involvement.

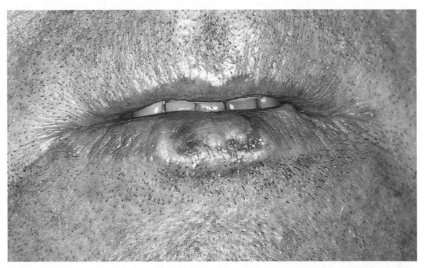

303 Diffuse carcinomatous change in the lower lip. This was a 'lip at risk', having been exposed to multiple courses of ultra violet radiation for a skin condition. (See Chapter 3.)

213

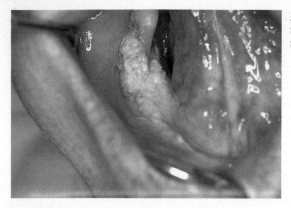

304 A verrucous carcinoma of the alveolar mucosa.

Salivary gland neoplasms

Ten per cent of all salivary gland neoplasms affect the minor salivary glands of the oral cavity. Of these the great majority (80%) occur in the palatal glands. The majority of these lesions are pleomorphic adenomas but more aggressive lesions, such as adenocystic carcinomas, may have precisely similar clinical characteristics, at least in the early stages. By and large pleomorphic adenomas are pain-free and slowly growing (**305**), but much more aggressive growth patterns may occur in some instances (**306** and **307**). Ulceration and rapid growth may be considered as possible markers of a malignant neoplasm, but the behaviour of the salivary tumours as a whole is unpredictable—such lesions should always be treated with suspicion, whatever their clinical characteristics.

305 A small pleomorphic adenoma in the palatal mucosa. In this case, the growth had been so slow as to have been mistaken for a static lesion and a denture constructed so as to avoid it.

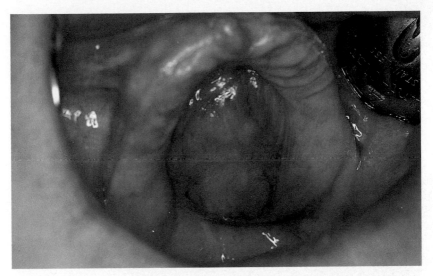

306 In contrast to the lesion shown in **306**, this is a rapidly growing pleomorphic adenoma, having been present for less than a year. Although the lesion was histologically non-malignant, it demonstrates the uncertain nature of histological prediction in the case of these lesions—the underlying palatal bone was infiltrated by tumour.

307 An adenocystic carcinoma in the palate. Although ulceration may be an indicator of malignant potential, it is an unreliable one.

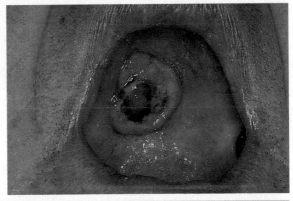

Salivary gland neoplasms

Diagnosis: Initially clinical, confirmed by biopsy. Form of biopsy (excisional or incisional?) remains controversial.

Melanoma

Intra-oral melanoma is a relatively rare lesion, but a very significant one in view of its highly aggressive characteristics. Early metastatic growth and fatal sequelae are common (**308**). The clinical recognition of an early melanoma and its differential diagnosis from a simple melanotic macule may be difficult, and the characteristic features of neoplastic growth—proliferation and rapid expansion—may occur after metastatic growth is established. Other melanotic lesions of the mucosa are discussed in Chapter 11.

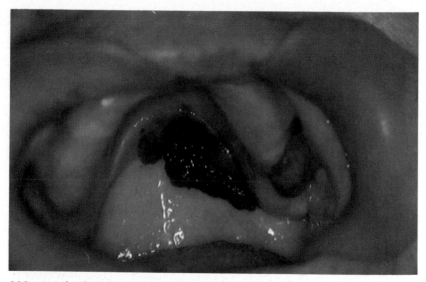

308 A palatal melanoma. Proliferative growth in a melanotic lesion should always be treated with grave suspicion.

Melanoma

Diagnosis: Opinions vary widely as to when and how to biopsy suspect melanoma. An expert opinion is essential. Important differential diagnoses: from other melanotic lesions (Chapter 11), from amalgam tattoo.

Other neoplasms

A wide range of neoplasms, both primary and secondary, may appear in the oral cavity, but these, however, are relatively uncommon compared to carcinoma. In particular, secondary neoplasms are rare, but there are many possible primary sources including the lungs, breasts and gastro-intestinal tract. The appearance of metastatic neoplastic tissue in abnormally healing, post-extraction tooth sockets has been described in a number of cases, as have metastatic neoplasms appearing in the form of an epulis. Such lesions may be difficult to identify on a clinical basis—histological assessment of the abnormal tissue may give the first indication of entirely unsuspected neoplasia. Other neoplasms may appear in the oral cavity as direct extensions from adjacent tissues, invading or expanding the oral mucosa (**309, 310** and **311**). The high incidence of oral lymphoma and Kaposi's sarcoma in HIV-positive individuals has been discussed in Chapter 1.

309 Carcinoma of the maxillary sinus invading the oral cavity—this was the first clinical manifestation of the neoplasm, although the lesion was well advanced (see **310**).

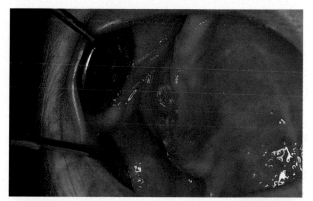

310 Radiograph of the patient shown in **309**—the right maxillary sinus is filled with tumour and the bony margins have been destroyed.

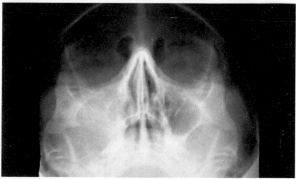

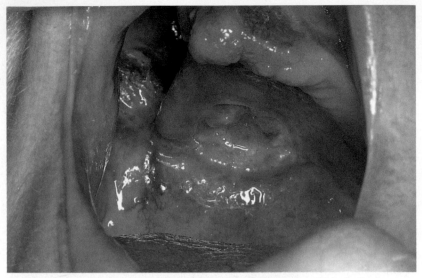

311 An osteosarcoma in the maxilla—an unusual site. This lesion was a post-operative recurrence following partial maxillectomy.

Haemangioma, papilloma

Haemangiomas—hamartomas rather than neoplasms—have been discussed under the heading of vascular lesions in Chapter 9. For reasons of clinical convenience, papillomas and related lesions have also been dealt with in Chapter 9.

Chapter 11

Endocrine Abnormalities, Mucosal Pigmentation and Drug-Related Conditions

Physiological endocrine changes

At times of unusual hormonal activity or change, in particular during pregnancy, the gingivae become unusually susceptible to inflammatory change. Characteristically, this results in a rather hyperplastic gingivitis, particularly affecting the papillae (**312**), which in a few cases may become localised so as to produce a 'pregnancy epulis' (**313**). The histology of these lesions is of a somewhat vascular immature granulation tissue and, occasionally, they may increase in size in an alarming manner. However, there is often virtually complete recession

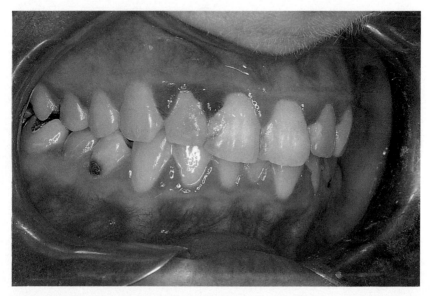

312 Pregnancy gingivitis. This is a characteristic but relatively mild case.

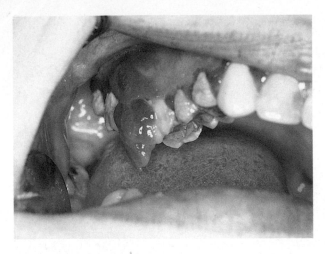

313 A pregnancy epulis—a single papilla has expanded to form the epulis in this otherwise quite mild pregnancy gingivitis.

with the end of pregnancy if excision has not been carried out. Strict oral hygiene will generally minimise the changes of pregnancy gingivitis, although there are wide variations in opinion as to the importance of the factors causing the condition. A similar, usually less marked, change may transiently occur during puberty, but again, opinions vary as to the relative significance of oral hygiene maintenance and also the effect of permanent tooth eruption. Many other conditions (for instance, the 'burning mouth syndrome') have been ascribed to hormonal changes of the menopause. There is little evidence for these suppositions.

Endocrine abnormalities

The oral mucosa may be affected in a number of endocrine abnormalities—in particular the endocrine—candidiasis syndrome (discussed in Chapter 1). By far the most common endocrine disorder leading to oral candidiasis (usually acute pseudomembranous) is diabetes mellitus—any patient presenting with unexplained oral candidiasis should undergo appropriate screening (**314**). It is also generally accepted that patents with diabetes melitus have an exaggerated tendency towards periodontal disease (**315**). However, just as in the case of 'pregnancy gingivitis' mentioned above, there is confusion as to the various factors which may be implicated in the periodontal changes.

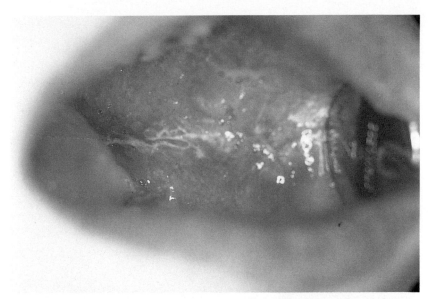

314 Pseudomembranous candidiasis (thrush) in a patient with poorly controlled diabetes.

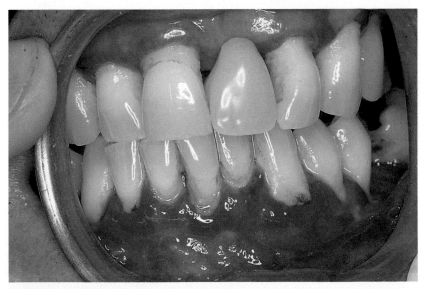

315 Periodontal disease in a diabetic patient.

Both hyper- and hypo-adrenocortical activity may lead to oral changes and, particularly, to candidiasis. In Addison's disease (autoimmune disruption of the adrenal cortex) mucocutaneous candidiasis may occur with either atrophic or pseudomembranous oral lesions (**316**, **317** and **318**). In addition, oral melanosis may be present (**319**)—the two together constitute a classic marker for Addison's disease (**320**). In hyperadrenocortical states (as in Cushing's syndrome), oral candidiasis is also common (**321**). An even rarer endocrine-dependent situation may arise in the oral medicine context. The abnormal bone growth associated with acromegaly (almost always the result of a pituitary tumour) may manifest itself either as a late-developing and progressive orthodontic abnormality (**322** and **323**) or in facial pain—the result of changing muscle/skeletal balance. Such a diagnosis is highly unlikely to be made on the results of a single oral examination.

Endocrine abnomalities

Diagnosis: Diagnosis of endocrine disorders is highly specialised. If suspected, referal to an endocrinologist is essential.

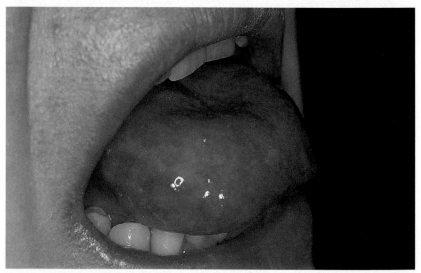

316 Atrophic candidiasis of the tongue in hypoadrenocorticalism (Addison's disease).

317 Candidal infection of the fingernails in the patient shown in **316**.

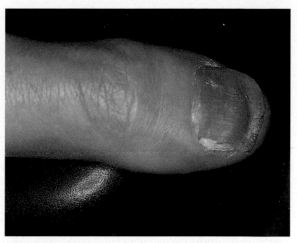

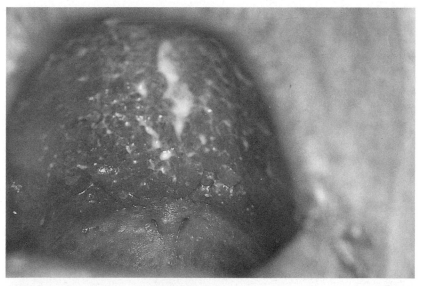

318 Pseudomem-branous candidiasis in previously undiagnosed Addison's disease.

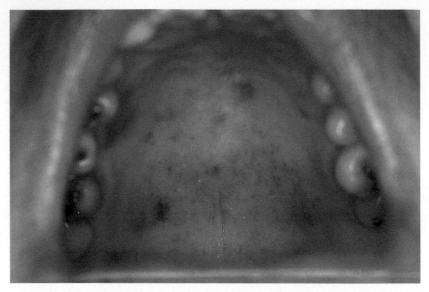

319 Melanotic pigmentation of the oral mucosa—often (as here) the first indication of Addison's disease.

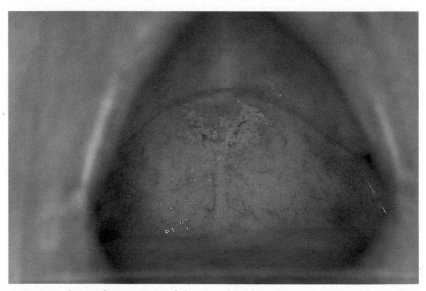

320 Pseudomembranous candidiais and melanotic pigmentation occurring together in Addison's disease.

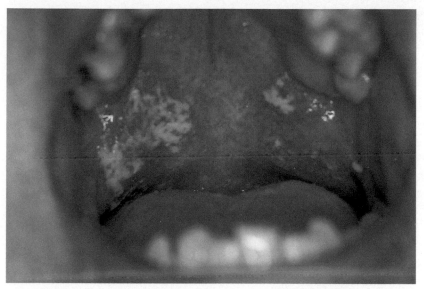

321 Hyperadrenocorticism (Cushing's syndrome). Widespread oral pseudomembranous candidiasis—the primary aetiological factor in this patient was an adrenal tumour causing a gross overproductionof natural corticosteroids.

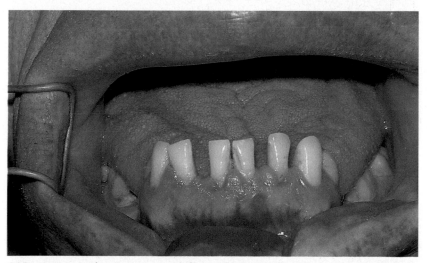

322 Acromegaly. Spacing and forward movement of the lower teeth in acromegaly—the tongue was greatly enlarged.

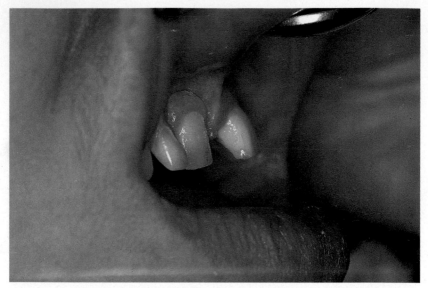

323 Bone growth in the maxilla of the patient shown in **321** demonstrated by the comparison of the position of the natural teeth with that on the partial denture, made two years previously. The earliest symptoms in this patient were of facial pain consistent with a diagnosis of temporomandibular joint disturbance—the result of renewed bone growth.

Mucosal pigmentation: melanosis

By far the most common reason for melanotic pigmentation of the oral mucosa is racial—the distribution is highly variable, but, in general, pigmented mucosa is an accompaniment of pigmented skin (**324**). In many cases, however, the mucosa alone (most commonly of the gingivae) may be involved. In a few patients, melanotic pigmentation may occur relatively rapidly and late in life, without any detectable systemic disturbance to account for this (**325**). In general, however, and as mentioned above, late-onset mucosal pigmentation should be considered as a possible sign of endocrine disturbance (see **Table 21,** page 228).

Single static melanotic patches of the mucosa—particularly of the lips—may be considered as simple melanotic macules. This is a diagnosis comparable to a skin freckle, and should always be made with awareness of the possible differential diagnoses (**326**). Drug-induced melanosis is well known but relatively rare. Reactive melanosis, occurring in the corium underlying the epithelium, either in lichen planus or in leukoplakia has been described in Chapter 7 (see Figure **177**).

The Peutz–Jegher syndrome is a rare condition in which oral, perioral and facial melanotic macules occur in association with multiple intestinal polyps. This is a genetically determined condition, transmitted as an autosomal dominant characteristic. There is no explanation for the strange association of lesions (**327** and **328**).

The major differential diagnosis of a melanotic patch of the oral mucosa is from amalgam pigmentation, which may occur in the most unlikely sites (**329**) and may be noticed only after many years when the significant history may have been forgotten. An amalgam patch may be quite undetectable on routine radiology, as the metallic content becomes widely dispersed in the tissues and effectively radiolucent. Occasionally, an inflamatory lesion with a haemorrhagic component may be mistaken for a melanotic lesion on superficial examination (**330**); however, a full clinical examination will, in general, correct this error.

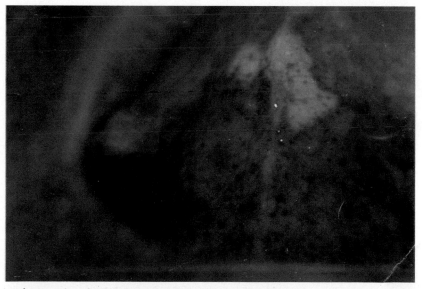

324 Racial melanotic pigmentation of the oral mucosa.

TABLE 21 Causes of Oral Melanosis	
Racial	
Endocrine disturbances	
	Addison's disease
	Cushing's syndrome
Reactive	
	Lichen planus
	Leukoplakia
Drug-related	
	Oral contraceptives
	Antimalarials
	Phenothiazines
	Methyldopa
	Many others reported

Important differential diagnosis: *From amalgam pigmentation.*

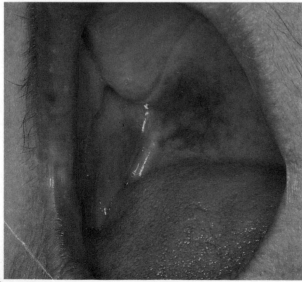

325 Diffuse melanotic pigmentation of the oral mucosa occurring in a middle-aged Caucasian patient. Despite intensive investigation, no cause for this was found.

326 Simple melanotic macules on the lower lip.

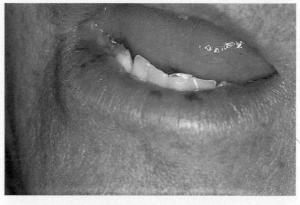

327 Peutz–Jeghers syndrome—circumoral melanotic macules. The patient is a 13-year-old female patient who had already had a partial gut resection for multiple polyps. Her father had a similar history.

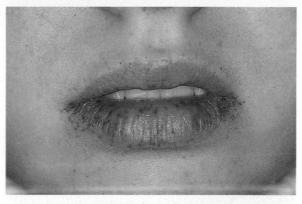

328 The secondary distribution of melanotic macules across the bridge of the nose in Peutz–Jeghers syndrome.

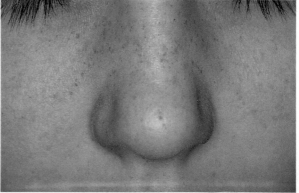

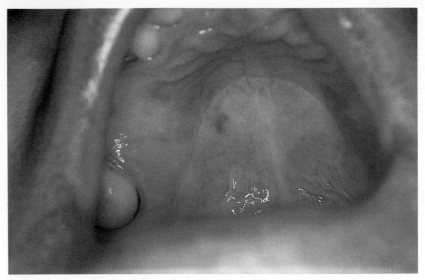

329 Amalgam pigmentation. This illustrates the sometimes unlikely sites in which amalgam may be deposited in the soft tissues, eventually to produce an amalgam 'tattoo'. This lesion was the long-term result of an accident with an amalgam gun in which the palatal musosa was breached.

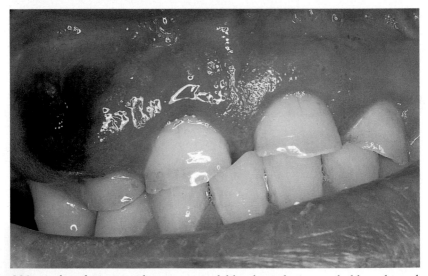

330 A dental sinus with extravasated blood producing a darkly coloured lesion which could be mistaken for a melanotic area.

Drug-related conditions

Chemical burns of the mucosa are not uncommon; they are usually the result either of accidental ingestion of the responsible agent (**331**) or of the unprotected use of caustic dental medicaments (**332**). The most common source of chemical burns in the mouth is the use of toothache remedies applied to the tooth or gingivae, the most common of which is aspirin (**333**) (see **Table 21**).

TABLE 21   Drug-Related Conditions of the Oral Mucosa*

Chemical burns

    Aspirin
    Toothache remedies
    Root canal medicaments
    Acids

Allergic reactions

    Penicillin
    Other antibiotics
    Eugenol
    Metals (rare)

Lichenoid reactions

Erythema multiforme
    (see **Table 13**)

Gingival hyperplasia

    Phenytoin
    Cyclosporin
    Nifedipine

Candidiasis

    Steroids
    Antibiotics
    Melanosis
        (see **Table 20**)

These are the most common conditions and the most frequently involved drugs, but many others have been reported.

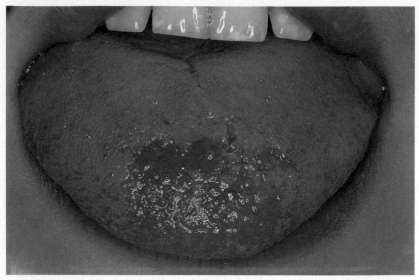

331 Chemical burn caused by the use of a pipette to transfer a dilute sodium hydroxide solution. The damage is mild—largely due to depapillation.

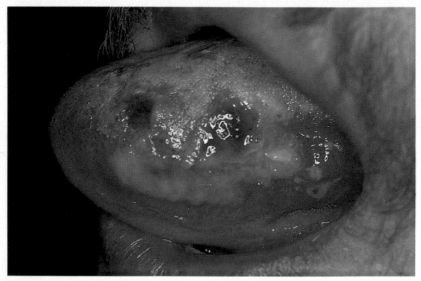

332 A more severe chemical burn caused by leakage of a root canal sterilizing agent maintained in contact for some time by the saliva isolation measures.

The oral cavity may be involved in a wide range of generalised (type 1) allergic reactions, most frequently to antibiotics (**334**). The resulting swelling of the tongue may require urgent action to relieve the airway in severe cases. Local contact (type 4) allergy may also occur in response to antibiotics (**335**) and from dental materials—eugenol is the most common, particularly in patients with established reactions to the essential oils in perfumes. Allergy to metals in denture bases is occasionally confirmed by patch testing, but is much less common than might be supposed. The same is true of allergy to plastisisers and other components of acrylic resins.

Antibiotics, used either locally or systemically, fairly frequently cause other oral problems—most commonly of 'antibiotic sore tongue' (**336**) or 'hairy tongue' (**337**). (See Chapter 3 for a discussion of hairy tongue.) These difficulties are significantly more frequent when antibiotic therapy is combined with steroid therapy—in these circumstances candida are virtually always involved (**338**). The problem of steroid-induced candidiasis has been discussed in Chapter 1 (see Figure **46**).

The lichenoid reaction and erythema multiforme precipitated by drugs (**339** and **340**) have been discussed in Chapter 7 and the most common drugs involved tabulated (see **Table 13**). Pemphigus-, pemphigoid- and lupus-like lesions have also been reported as drug-induced conditions although these are much less common then lichenoid reactions. An equally wide range of drugs has been implicated.

Exfoliative stomatitis is not unusual during the treatment of malignancy or other conditions with cytotoxic drugs. This may range from a relatively minor condition (**341**) to one causing a great deal of discomfort (**342**).

Gingival hyperplasia is an established side effect of treatment with phenytoin, cyclosporin and calcium channel blocking agents (**343** and **344**). The essential mechanism is of proliferation and hyperactivity of fibroblasts in the connective tissue component of the gingivae. In some cases, particularly in the case of cyclosporin, the changes may be gross and rapidly progressive (**345**). The gingival enlargement is characteristically papillary in nature. As in the case of other gingival abnormalities there is uncertainty as to the significance of the role of oral hygiene in the progress of these hyperplastic conditions.

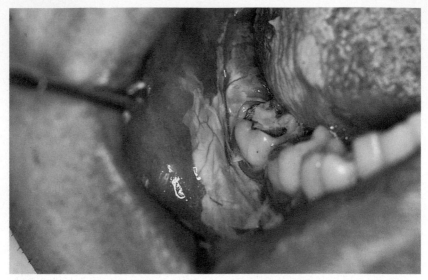

333 An aspirin burn caused by dissolving a single tablet of aspirin on the buccal mucosa adjoining an aching tooth. The sudden appearance of an acute leukoplakia-like lesion associated with a history of toothache in the area should always be considered as possibly being the result of the use of toothache remedies.

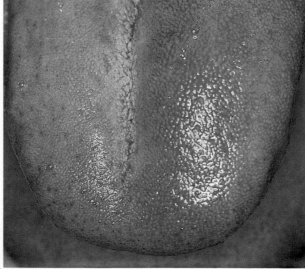

334 An oral reaction to penicillin is relatively uncommon. In this patient, undergoing a generalised penicillin reaction (type 1), there is unilateral oedema of the tongue.

335 A mild vesicular contact allergic reaction (type 4) to tetracycline used as a mouthwash.

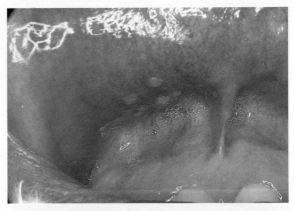

336 An 'antibiotic sore tongue' following tetracycline therapy. There are some areas of filliform atrophy and some other brown somewhat 'hairy' patches.

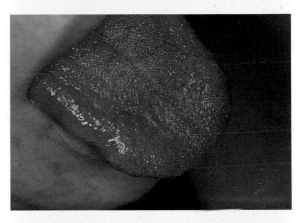

337 A 'black hairy tongue' following a course of systemic tetracycline therapy for a respiratory infection.

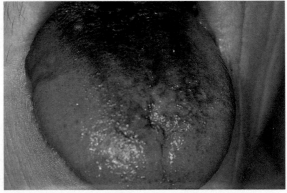

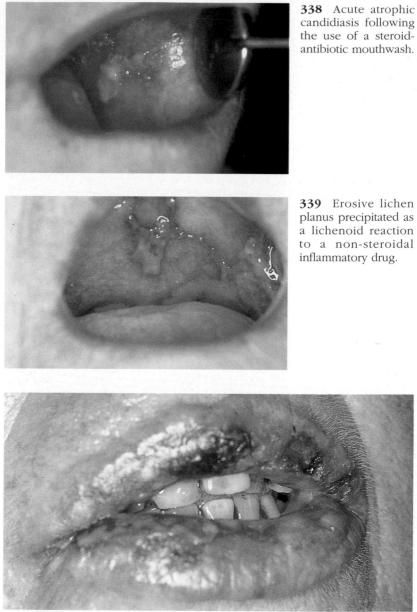

338 Acute atrophic candidiasis following the use of a steroid-antibiotic mouthwash.

339 Erosive lichen planus precipitated as a lichenoid reaction to a non-steroidal inflammatory drug.

340 Erythema multiforme; also a reaction to a non-steroidal inflammatory agent.

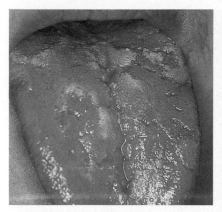

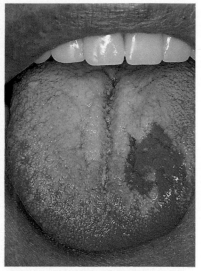

341 Depapillation of the tongue, resembling a geographic tongue but causing much more discomfort, in a patient prescribed azathioprine for severe oro-genital ulceration. The depapillation was reversed on withdrawal of the azathioprine.

342 A painful glossitis, with patchy depapillation, in a patient taking cytotoxic drugs for control of cervical metasteses of an oral carcinoma.

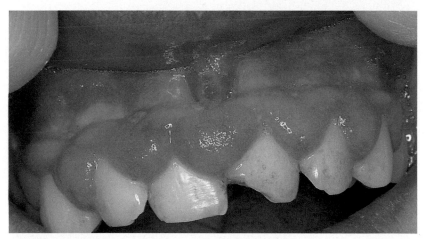

343 Phenytoin (epanutin)-induced hyperplastic gingivitis. This shows the characteristic appearance of the condition with individual enlargement of the interdental papillae. In later stages, and in the absence of treatment, secondary inflammatory changes may intervene and the texture of the gingivae may become much less firm.

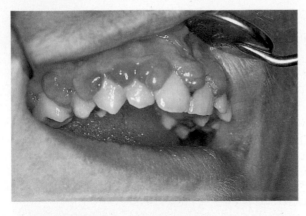

344 Gingival hyperplasia associated with cyclosporin in a renal transplant patient. This is in a relatively early phase.

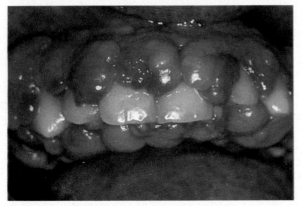

345 Gross gingival hyperplasia, also associated with the use of cyclosporin in a renal transplant patient.

Drug-related conditions

Diagnosis: Attempted confirmation of suspect allergy by challenge to be undertaken only by specialists in hospital conditions. Anapylaxis is a possibility.

Chapter 12

Teeth and Supporting Bone

The teeth

The teeth are stable structures, and play virtually no part in metabolic disease after their final calcification and eruption. It follows that the teeth represent the condition of the patient at the time of calcification. There are, however, a large number of recognised conditions in which abnormalities in structure, morphology or pattern of eruption of the teeth are genetically linked to abnormalities of bone or other epidermal structures. In erupted teeth (and with the exception of caries), only those conditions which lead to loss of tooth substance— erosion, abrasion and attrition—significantly affect their appearance.

The size of the teeth is genetically determined and, in general, significant variation from the norm is an isolated abnormality, not linked to generalised growth disorders or to any form of systemic disease (**346**). Teeth missing from their normal place in the dental arch could have been extracted, may be congenitally absent or could be unerupted. Congenital absence of some of the teeth (hypodontia or partial anodontia) may be a purely local condition with no systemic manifestations, or may represent one manifestation of a complex syndrome as mentioned above. Total anodontia is extremely rare. Abnormal tooth morphology may represent an individual variation, or may be associated with hypodontia or with complex syndromes (**347**). On the whole, delayed tooth eruption is not associated with endocrine abnormalities, although there are a few genetically determined (non-endocrine–based) disorders in which delayed eruption of the teeth is a feature (**348** and **349**). In Down's syndrome, the teeth may be of abnormal morphology or size, but this is an inconstant finding.

Dental and enamel hypoplasia

Hypoplasia of the dental tissues is also a multifactorial condition. Disturbances of either enamel or dentine may occur, often in combination, resulting either from faulty matrix formation or from defective calcification mechanisms. The terms 'amelogenesis imperfecta', 'enamel hypocalcification' and 'dentinogenesis imperfecta' are rather loosely used to describe these abnormalities. The disturbances of dentine formation are less clearly defined than those of enamel. These

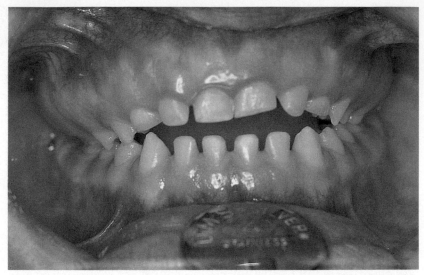

346 Microdontia—what appear to be deciduous teeth in this 16-year-old patient are in fact unusually small permanent teeth. There was no other detectable associated abnormality. Compare with **349**, which shows multiple retained deciduous teeth.

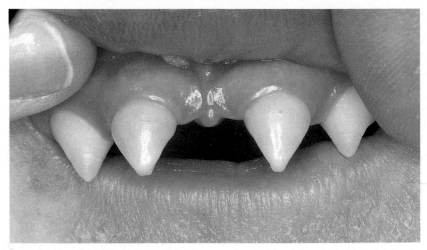

347 Hypodontia. Peg-shaped permanent incisors in a patient with anhydrotic ectodermal dysplasia. An isolated peg-shaped tooth (often an upper lateral incisor) in an otherwise normal dentition is common and of no other diagnostic significance.

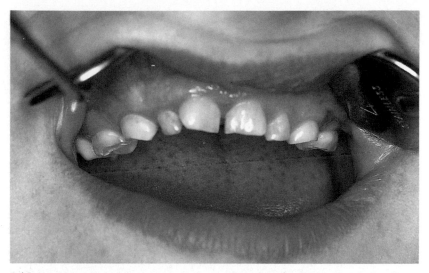

348 Retained deciduous teeth in a patient with cleidocranial dysplasia (dysostosis). In this condition defective membrane bone formation affecting the clavicle and frontal bone is associated with the presence of multiple supernumerary teeth which often remain unerupted (see **349**). This is perhaps the best known of the complex conditions in which abnormalities of the teeth are associated with abnormal bone formation.

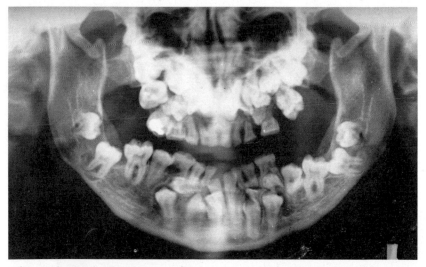

349 Radiograph of patient in **348** showing multiple unerupted teeth.

hypoplasias may be either hereditary (**350**, **351** and **352**), or the result of infantile disease or metabolic disturbances (**353**, **354**, **355** and **356**). The forms of dentinal and enamel hypoplasia and associated factors are summarised in **Table 22** and **Table 23** .

TABLE 22   Hypoplasia of Enamel and Dentine*

Acquired conditions due to:

> Local infection
> Generalised infection
> Generalised metabolic disease
> Trophic disturbances
> > (including prenatal and neonatal)
> Endocrine disorders (inconsistent)
> Fluorosis

Developmental conditions

> Amelogenisis imperfecta
> Hypoplastic type (matrix defect)
> Hypocalcification
> Dentinogenisis imperfecta
> Dentine only
> With osteogenisis imperfecta

In acquired conditions either enamel or dentine may be involved, depending on degree of tooth development at time of influencing factor.

350 Amelogenesis imperfecta—hypocalcified type. The poorly calcified enamel can be seen flaking away from the underlying dentine.

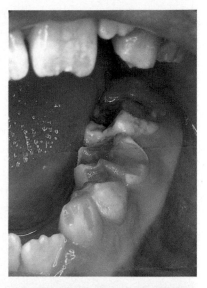

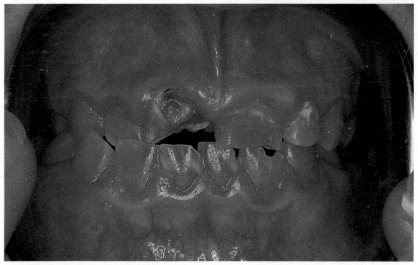

351 Dentinogenesis imperfecta. The poorly formed dentine gives the teeth a characteristically opalescent appearance—hence the term 'hereditary opalescent dentine' This may be the only defect present but, in some patients, may be associated with osteogenesis imperfecta (see **352**). Several classifications of dentinogenesis imperfecta have been suggested, largely based on the associated conditions.

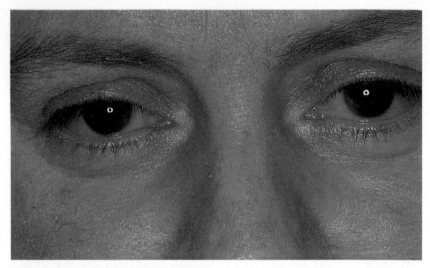

352 This is a member of a family of whom all showed dentinogenesis imperfecta, varying degrees of osteogenesis imperfecta and the blue sclera characteristic of osteogenesis imperfecta.

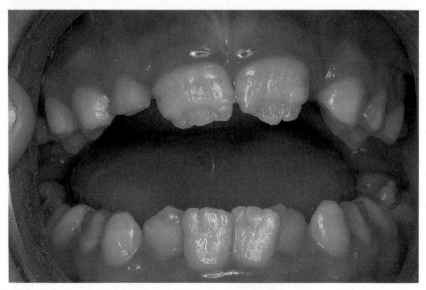

353 Band-like distribution of hypoplastic enamel at the incisal edge of the upper central incisors. The patient had a severe febrile illness within the first year of life.

TABLE 24   Hypoplasia of Enamel and Dentine: Systemic Factors*

Prenatal	Infections —e.g. rubella, syphilis Gross maternal metabolic disturbance
Neonatal	Hypocalcaemia Severe neonatal hypoxia Severe hyperbilirubinaemia (infantile jaundice)
Infantile	Malnutrition G.I. tract disease (e.g. Coeliac disease) Infections Endocrine disorders Fluorosis

Dental hypoplasia has been described in occasional association with a wide range of conditions both acquired and developmental.

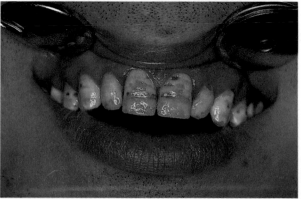

354 Generalised enamel hypoplasia with pitting and staining characteristic of fluorosis. The patient was born and spent his early childhood in a Mediterranean area having extremely high natural fluoride content in the drinking water.

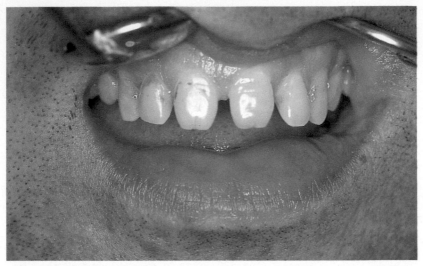

355 Hypoplastic enamel and abnormal tooth morphology in a patient with congenital syphilis. This is the classical manifestation—Hutchinson's incisors (barrel-shaped and notched in the centre of the incisal edge).

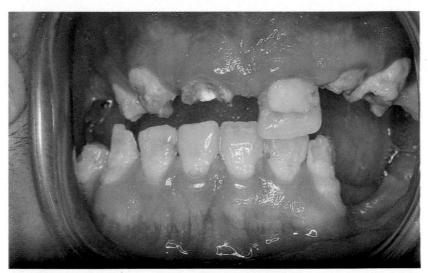

356 Hypocalcification of both enamel and dentine in a patient with a gross infantile abnormality of calcium absorption. The bones were also affected. Such gross calcium deficiencies are rare as a cause of dental abnormalities.

Discolouration of the teeth

Discolouration of the teeth may occur in a few infantile diseases, but the most common cause of widespread tooth discolouration remains tetracycline staining (**357** and **358**). This, of course, has now become very unusual in new patients, due to the almost complete abandonment of the use of such antibiotics in childhood and pregnancy. However, extrinsic stains may be acquired, as may intrinsic discolouration of individual teeth, usually the result of trauma.

Loss of tooth substance by abrasion and erosion have been mentioned above. Abnormal degrees of abrasion (usually by tooth brushing), although not diagnostic, may be an indication of a somewhat obsessive behaviour pattern (**359**). Loss of enamel by acid erosion, formerly considered only to be an industrial hazard, is now considered much more likely to be found in patients with a high consumption of acid drinks (including some fruit juice preparations) (**360**). It may also be a marker of regular vomiting or regurgitation—it is a common finding in bulimic patients.

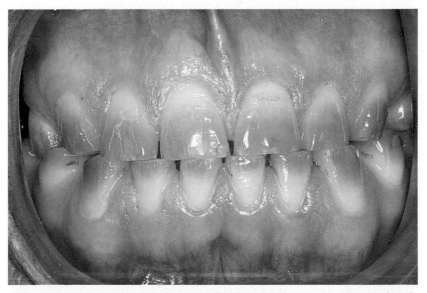

357 Tetracycline staining—as is usually the case this is not associated with any evident hypoplastic changes—compare with **356**.

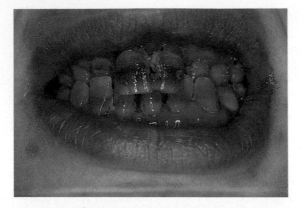

358 Severe tetracycline staining associated with hypoplastic enamel. It is thought that in such cases the hypoplasia is the result of the primary disease process rather than of the tetracycline.

Discolouration

Diagnosis: Clinical, radiographic.

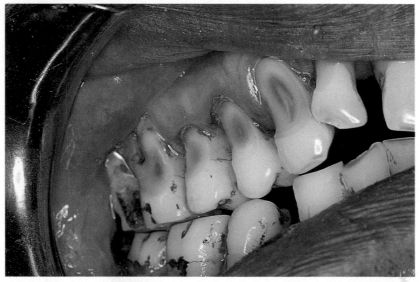

359 Severe toothbrush abrasion which has penetrated to the former pulp chambers of the teeth, now filled by secondary dentine. There is also evidence of attrition—wearing away of the teeth by contact with each other. There is tobacco staining of the exposed dentine and leukoedema of the buccal mucosa.

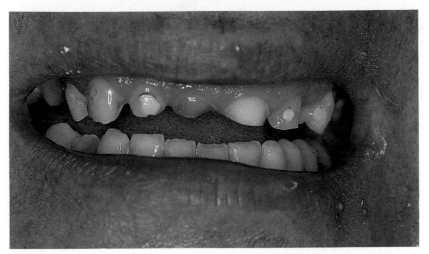

360 Erosion—in this case, the result of drinking large quantities of a soft drink with a very acid pH.

Lesions of supporting bone

A wide range of lesions of the bone may be seen in and around the jaws, but the vast majority of these are of inflammatory origin (for example, dental cysts) or are relatively simple bone overgrowths and exostoses (**361**). There are, however, two dystrophic conditions of bone which are seen from time to time in the jaws and may present for diagnosis. These are monostotic fibrous dysplasia (**362** and **363**) and Paget's disease (**364, 365** and **366**). Other dystrophic or metabolic bone diseases (including polyostotic fibrous dysplasia) present only very rarely for diagnosis as a result of oral manifestations. It is evident that, from time to time, neoplasms of bone may occur in the jaws and initially appear with intra-oral manifestations (**367**).

Lesions of supporting bone

Diagnosis: Monostotic fibrous dysplasia: clinical, radiological, biopsy (may be difficult because of haemorrhage), blood chemistry normal.

Paget's disease: Clinical, radiological, blood chemistry abnormal (alkaline phosphatase–elevated; other biochemical tests available).

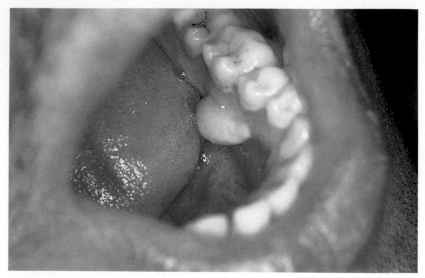

361 A simple bony outgrowth of the mandible in a characteristic site—the so-called torus mandibularis. Other similar lesions may be seen in the midline of the hard palate (torus palatinus). They are static and completely benign.

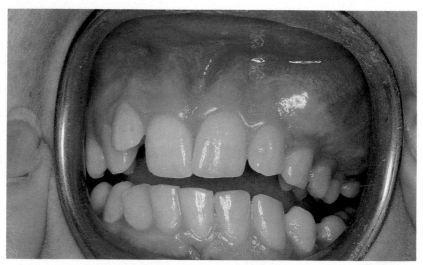

362 Monostotic fibrous dysplasia of the maxilla in a 16-year-old patient. As is usually the case, this was an isolated lesion and (as is always the case) the blood chemistry was normal. A radiograph is shown in **363**.

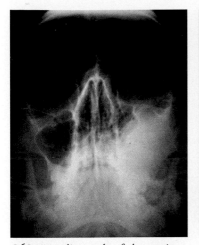

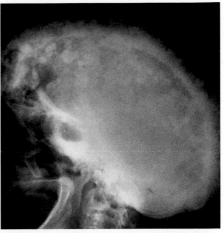

363 A radiograph of the patient shown in **362**. There is obliteration of the maxillary sinus by the bone growth of the fibrous dysplasia.

364 Paget's disease—a radiograph illustrating the more usual situation of widespread bony changes throughout the skull. It is a common condition in elderly patients and in most cases is symptom-free and not discovered except as an incidental finding. Ill-fitting dentures may be the patient's complaint—the maxilla may be slowly expanding, the mandible less likely so.

365 In a few patients, the areas of Pagetoid bone may be relatively circumscribed—in this case to two dense masses in the maxilla (see **366**).

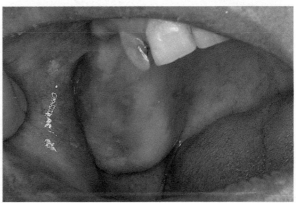

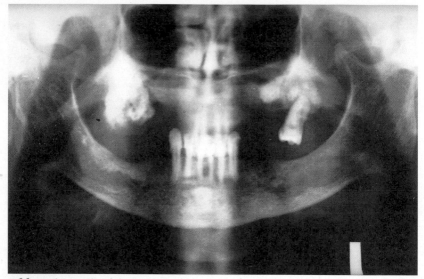

366 Radiograph of the patient shown in **365** demonstrating bilateral areas of abnormally dense bone in the maxilla.

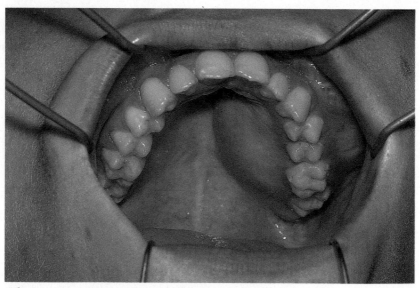

367 An osteosarcoma of the maxilla in a young female patient. It had grown to the size illustrated without any pain or other marked symptoms.

Index

skin diseases, 115
  bullous, 129–50
  lichen planus, 115–28
smoker's keratosis, 199, 202
solar keratosis, 78
squamous cell carcinoma *see* carcinoma,
  oral
Staphylococcus aureus, 28, 74
steroids, 39, 40
Stevens–Johnson syndrome, 143
stomatitis, 31, 80, 233
syphilis, 34–6, 246
systemic lupus erythematosus, 152, 154–5,
  159
systemic sclerosis, 152, 157–8, 159

teeth, 239–49
  abrasion, 247, 248
  delayed eruption, 239, 241
  discolouration, 247–8
temporomandibular joint, 151, 153, 226
thrombocytopenia, 92–4
thrush, 21, 22–3, 40, 42, 43, 81
tobacco, 190, 192, 199, 200–1, 208, 212, 248
tongue, 40, 59–73
  carcinoma, 210
  chemical burn, 232
  crenated, 63
  depapillation, 65–6, 80, 83
  drug-induced changes, 234, 237
  erythema multiforme, 144
  fissuring, 59–60, 61–2
  geographic, 67–9
  hairy, 64, 235
  herpetiform ulceration, 56
  leukoplakia, 80, 82, 191, 192
  lichen planus, 119, 120, 123, 124, 125
  midline fissure, 109
  midline glossitis, 69–72
  primary herpetic stomatitis, 8–9, 10, 11
  primary syphilitic lesion, 35
  sarcoidosis, 111
  scrotal, 63
  sore, 72–3, 80
  tie *see* ankyloglossia
toothache remedies, 231, 234
torus mandibularis, 250
transplant procedures, 39, 40
Treponema pallidum, 34
trigeminal nerve, 15, 16
tuberculoid granuloma, 103, 104, 105, 108
tuberculosis, 37–8
tylosis, 203, 204, 205

ulceration, 17, 18, 45, 80
  see also oral ulceration, recurrent
ulcerative colitis, 96, 98–102

varicosities, 184–5
vascular lesions, 184–8
verruca, 20
Vincent's organisms, 32, 40
viral infections, 7, 45, 128
viral warts, 181–2
vitamin B12, 79
  deficiency, 83–6

Wegener's granulomatosis, 112–113
white sponge naevus *see* leukokeratosis

xerostomia, 45, 161–2, 164